IS THIS NORMAL?

THE ESSENTIAL GUIDE
TO MIDDLE AGE AND BEYOND

JOHN WHYTE, MD, MPH
CHIEF MEDICAL EXPERT FOR THE DISCOVERY CHANNEL

FOREWORD BY DEAN ORNISH, MD

RODAL

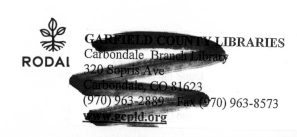

Rodale books may be purchased for business or promotional use or for special sales. For information, please write to:
Special Markets Department, Rodale Inc., 733 Third Avenue, New York, NY 10017

Printed in the United States of America
Rodale Inc. makes every effort to use acid-free ♾, recycled paper ♻.

Illustrations by Judy Newhouse
Book design by Christopher Rhoads

Library of Congress Cataloging-in-Publication Data

Whyte, John
.   Is this normal? : the essential guide to middle age and beyond / John Whyte.
        p.   cm.
    Includes index.
    ISBN 978–1–60961–450–8   paperback
    1. Middle-aged persons—Health and hygiene.   2. Aging.   I. Title.
RA777.5.W49   2011
613'.0434—dc22   2011012146

Distributed to the trade by Macmillan
2   4   6   8   10   9   7   5   3   1   paperback

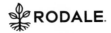

We inspire and enable people to improve their lives and the world around them.

rodalebooks.com

*To my mother, may we all age
as gracefully as you.*

CONTENTS

FOREWORD

A patient once told me, "Growing old is a bitch!" But it doesn't have to be.

The latest research reveals that our bodies are much more dynamic than once thought. Because of this, we're learning that diseases and conditions that used to be viewed as a normal part of aging can often be prevented and sometimes even reversed by making comprehensive lifestyle changes. These findings are giving many people new hope and new choices.

If you're from the baby boom generation, you're probably already inundated with books about how to care for your aging parents, how to marshal your financial resources for retirement, and what to do with all that spare time you'll supposedly have on your hands.

Taking care of your aging parents can certainly be a challenge, but learning to cope with the changes going on in your own body and mind can be even more disconcerting. If you're one of the 78 million baby boomers in the US anxiously awaiting the start of physical and mental changes, you may be wishing for a guidebook to see you through, and here it is.

Many people are embarrassed to bring concerns about every-day health challenges to their doctors or even to ask for advice from family and friends. What will happen to your skin, your joints, your metabolism, your eyes, your memory? What about relationships and sex (not to mention your bowels)?

Many accept health problems as just part of aging, because they do not realize that these problems are often preventable or treatable. They may live with pain, depression, failing eyesight, urinary incontinence, sexual dysfunction, and other difficulties that affect quality of life, because they believe these problems are normal. They may think it's inevitable that they will get heart disease, arthritis, osteoporosis, or cancer of the breast or prostate.

Is This Normal? is the guidebook middle-aged and older adults need. It explains what happens as you age, including how and why your body changes and what differences you can expect to your memory, emotions, physical functions, and relationships. It will alert you to changes that are definitely not normal, helping you know when you should seek medical care. And it will make clear that, whatever changes you are experiencing, you are not alone.

This book addresses your interest in looking and feeling younger. Thanks to medical research, we now know that some of the changes we used to take for granted—like weight gain, joint decay, and weakening muscles—can be reduced or prevented by a program of healthy eating and exercise. By explaining the science behind common age-related changes, *Is This Normal?* will help you make smart decisions about which antiaging treatments are likely to work and which ones are expensive snake oil.

Because about 4 out of 10 adults in the US now use some form of complementary and alternative medicine (CAM), this guidebook discusses the most reliable, scientifically proven treatments. CAM includes a group of diverse medical and health care systems, practices, and products that are not generally considered part of conventional medicine—from acupuncture and chiropractic to meditation, massage, and deep-breathing techniques. Many of these therapies and remedies are less costly than mainstream medical treatments as well, and you will learn how to make them a part of your system of self-care. This book offers an integrative approach, combining the best of conventional and complementary medicine.

Is This Normal? lets readers know not only whether the changes they are experiencing are normal, but also whether they need to see a physician or can treat minor ailments themselves. By offering crucial guidance for this stage of life, *Is This Normal?* addresses a widespread, unmet need. It offers information to help you navigate the changes of aging and arms you to face your fifties, sixties, seventies, and beyond with energy, health, and joy.

Dr. John Whyte, the Discovery Channel's chief medical expert, brings a unique perspective and state-of-the-art information. How well we live is as important as how long we live. Dr. Whyte shows us how we can do both.

Dean Ornish, MD
founder and president,
Preventive Medicine Research Institute, www.pmri.org;
clinical professor of medicine,
University of California, San Francisco;
and author of The Spectrum *and*
Dr. Dean Ornish's Program for Reversing Heart Disease

Chapter 1

ON THE OUTSIDE

True or False

There's nothing you can do to improve the look of wrinkles.   _____

As you age, you don't sweat as much.   _____

You don't need sunscreen as you get older.   _____

Everybody loses some hair with age.   _____

(Answers at end of chapter)

What do you know about your skin? I bet you didn't know it is the body's largest organ! (I'll let you in on a secret: Medical school professors always ask medical students, "What's the body's largest organ?" There's always a lot of giggling and even some blushing until they hear the answer.) On one level, the role of skin is pretty simple: It helps protect your internal organs from the outside environment. It also allows you to handle many things that are dirty or dangerous—like a baby's soiled diaper or that scary container in the back of the fridge—without worrying that germs will get into your bloodstream.

There's a lot more to your skin, though, than just keeping the germs out. For instance, skin helps you maintain your body temperature. It contains your sweat glands, which cool you down in the summer and keep heat in on a chilly winter day. Your skin

1

plays a big part in maintaining fluid balance, too. You might have heard that burn victims need huge amounts of fluid to keep them alive; that's because their skin has become so damaged that it can't keep enough water inside their bodies to maintain organ function.

Skin also alerts us to what's going on in the outside world. You might not have eyes in the back of your head, but I bet you know when someone is standing behind you and literally breathing down your neck. The nerve endings in your skin also warn you when the stove is hot, let you know that your drink needs ice even before you taste it, and tell you when it has just started to rain.

As you age, your skin undergoes a lot of changes. Some of these changes are inevitable, but others are preventable or can at least be delayed for a while. When it comes to age-related skin changes, wrinkles are the first issue that comes to mind for most people. But wrinkles are only one effect of our skin's aging process; as we approach middle age and beyond, our skin will undergo changes in texture, strength, and resilience. You're going to see some new spots and bumps. Some of these are more bothersome than dangerous, while others should send you right to the doctor. In other words, some changes are a normal part of aging, and some are not.

Don't panic. While wrinkles may be inevitable, getting older doesn't have to be a disaster for your skin. Knowing what to expect can help you take steps to protect your skin and keep it healthy as it ages with you.

STRUCTURE OF THE SKIN

Your skin is made up of three layers:

- Epidermis
- Dermis
- Hypodermis

Knowing a little bit about the functions of these layers and what they contain will help you understand the normal changes that come with aging as well as what you can do to keep your skin looking and feeling healthy.

Epidermis

The epidermis is the top layer—the one you see every day. The cells in this layer are renewed constantly, with the whole cycle of renewal taking about a month. That's right—you basically get a whole new layer of skin every month. Most of the cells in your epidermis are keratinocytes, which are largely dedicated to protecting the more sensitive, deeper layers of skin. These cells create a barrier against the elements, holding in fluids and protecting us

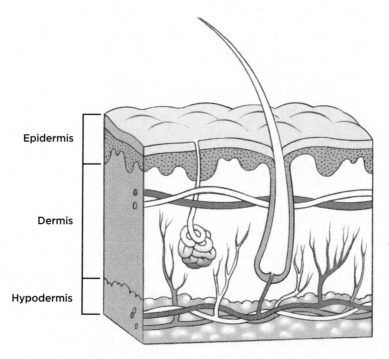

Epidermis

Dermis

Hypodermis

Cross section of the human skin.

against dangerous bacteria and viruses. The epidermis also contains melanocytes, the cells that give your skin its color.

Dermis

The next layer is the dermis. It holds blood vessels that feed the skin and nerves that carry sensations from it. Pressure, pain, and temperature are all recognized here. It also contains your oil glands and hair follicles. The dermis contains an important molecule called hyaluronic acid, which holds on to water to keep skin looking full and even. (We'll come back to hyaluronic acid in a little while.)

The dermis also contains collagen and elastin, two molecules that are essential to the appearance of your skin.

- **Collagen** allows skin to withstand physical stress without breaking or tearing. It also makes up most of the skin's mass. Without collagen, your skin would be a lot thinner and more easily damaged.
- **Elastin** does what it sounds like: It contributes elasticity to the skin. It lets skin "bounce back" from pressure and from everyday bumps and collisions. Think of elastin as a new crisp, tight rubber band.

Hypodermis

Underneath the dermis is the hypodermis. "Hypo" is derived from Greek and usually means "low" or "insufficient." But in anatomical terms, "hypo" means "below" or "under." Therefore the hypodermis is below the dermis. This layer contains a lot of fat cells to help cushion your skin and protect you from injury. These cells also serve as insulation, to help keep your body warm.

Why Wrinkles?

When it comes to wrinkles, everyone's different. Your genetic background has a big impact on how your skin will age. If your parents and grandparents had wrinkles in their fifties and sixties, chances are you will as well. I know America is all about fairness, but some people are just genetically gifted!

Genes aren't the only reason you get wrinkles, though. One of the biggest factors for premature aging is the amount of time you've spent in the sun over the years. When we were younger, of course, we thought a suntan made us look healthy and sexy. But as we get older, we pay a price for that mistaken belief. Sun-related aging, which doctors call photoaging, is superimposed on top of your natural aging process. So if you spent a lot of time at the beach working on your tan in your younger years, you will develop wrinkles sooner than your friends who stayed in the shade.

You might have noticed that people with naturally dark skin often seem to have fewer wrinkles than those with fair skin. That's because high levels of pigment protect their skin from sun damage. Naturally dark skin, however, is not the same as dark skin from tanning.

Did you ever wonder why your face seems to be the main place wrinkles appear? It feels like a cruel joke, but there's a reason your face ages first: Your facial muscles move your skin around a lot, causing folds and creases to appear and disappear. All of that folding and creasing puts stress on your skin, and eventually those temporary creases become permanent (so your mother was right—if you make "that expression," your face really will freeze that way). Aging and sun damage contribute to the process by decreasing the skin's ability to rebound. Most other muscles in your body serve to move your bones, like when you bend your knees or pick something up with your hands.

Though we all worry about gaining fat, as we get older, we actually *lose* fat in the hypodermis. Along with changes to collagen and elastin, this loss of fat contributes to the sagging of skin that used to look smooth and resilient.

THE SURFACE OF THE SKIN

In addition to gaining a few wrinkles, the look and feel of your skin changes as you age. Aging skin contains less water and lipids than younger skin. Lipids consist of fats, oils, waxes, and similar substances produced in your body. Without them, your epidermis could not do its job as a barrier to the outside world. As we get older, we have fewer lipids in the outermost layer of our skin, which means we cannot hold on to water as well, and therefore we develop drier skin. Certain lipids in the top layer of the epidermis help prevent unwanted bacteria from multiplying.

Our skin also produces less sebum as we age—the stuff that clogged your pores as a teenager and caused you to break out. At the same time, the renewal of skin cells in your epidermis no longer works as smoothly as it used to. All these factors combine to make skin drier and rougher as you get older.

Have you ever noticed that your or an elderly family member's skin appears thinner or even translucent? That's also a normal part of aging, and it's made more noticeable because the blood vessels beneath the skin's surface are becoming more visible.

Our skin becomes more delicate as we age. A scrape or bump that would lead to a minor scratch on younger skin can actually cause older skin to tear, almost like a piece of tissue paper. That's because the epidermis and dermis have become more fragile, and loss of elastin decreases the skin's ability to bounce back from impact. That once fresh, tight rubber band begins to get a little stretched out over the years.

Have you noticed that you seem to sweat less these days? That's a skin change, too. As we age, the output from our sweat glands declines; this may be one reason why older adults tend to be at a higher risk of heat stroke in the summer than younger folks. When we don't sweat as much, our bodies can overheat easily. It's important for older adults to drink plenty of fluids when they're exposed to extreme heat to prevent overheating.

SUN EXPOSURE AND SMOKING

My generation didn't think much about sunscreen when we were kids, and I'm sure we're paying for it now. I wouldn't be surprised if today's children, who get slathered with SPF 50 before setting foot on the beach, have different experiences with their skin as they age. But for those of us who had a suntan every summer for most of our younger lives, sun damage is a big deal.

One of the things that happens when you get a suntan is that ultraviolet (UV) radiation from the sun causes molecules called free radicals to form in your skin. Free radicals interact readily with other molecules in your body, altering their structures. Reactions caused by free radicals damage collagen and elastin, and slow down the production of new collagen. Damage from free radicals is part of normal aging, so there's no way to avoid it completely. But staying out of the sun and wearing sunscreen when you do go outside will definitely help protect you from the worst effects of UV rays.

The sun produces two types of radiation that you need protection from: ultraviolet A and ultraviolet B rays. They're abbreviated UVA and UVB, and that's what you'll see on your sunscreen label. (There's actually a UVC as well, but the ozone layer blocks most of it out.) UVB radiation, which is mostly absorbed in the epidermis, is the main cause of sunburns. Exposure to UVB radiation also

contributes to aging and can cause skin cancer. UVA light pene-
trates more easily into the dermis. It also ages your skin. Both
UVA and UVB light can cause lasting damage, so look for sun-
screens with UVA and UVB protection and a sun protection factor (SPF) of at least 15. Higher SPF numbers provide more
protection but not typically much more. I recommend SPF 15
because it protects against about 93 percent of UVB rays; SPF
30 protects against 97 percent. I often see people buying sunscreen with a high SPF like 60, mistakenly thinking that it will
protect them enough to stay outside all day. It won't. SPF 60 is not
twice as powerful as SPF 30.

And when the sunscreen bottle says to reapply after 2 hours?
Do it. It's not a marketing ploy to get you to buy more sunscreen.
Sunscreen does wear off, especially when you sweat. And some of
the ingredients may actually become less effective the longer
they're exposed to sunlight.

I get a lot of questions nowadays about vitamin D and sunscreen. Your body makes vitamin D when your skin is exposed to
UVB light. And we need vitamin D for all kinds of things: It helps
keep our bones strong, our immune systems working, and our
kidneys, liver, and thyroid gland functioning properly. The logical
next question is if we're limiting our exposure to the sun by using
sunscreen, should we take vitamin D supplements? The reality is
that you probably don't need more than half an hour of exposure
to the midday sun, a couple of times a week, in order for your
body to make enough vitamin D.[1] You can also get vitamin D
from the foods you eat—common grocery items such as milk
and cereal are fortified with vitamin D, and fish such as tuna
and mackerel are natural sources of the vitamin. If you do
choose to take a daily supplement, I usually recommend a dosage of 400 to 600 IU per day. Don't go much above this; higher
doses can be dangerous.

If you're considering taking a vitamin D supplement, be

aware of your local climate: If you live in the northern United States, winter sunlight might not be strong enough to trigger vitamin D production. Dark-skinned individuals may also need some supplementation.

In addition to sun exposure, smoking is another lifestyle choice that can affect your skin. In fact, premature skin aging due to smoking even has a name: it's called smokers' wrinkles.[2]

Why does a smoker's skin age faster? Because all of that smoke comes into contact with the top layer of the skin, and it causes irritation. Smoking also affects blood circulation, including the blood that feeds skin. And the movements that go along with smoking—pursing lips around that cigarette—can create creases that eventually become wrinkles. The moral of the story is—you guessed it—don't smoke.

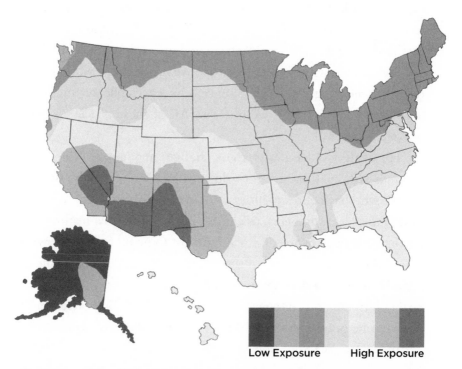

Low Exposure   High Exposure

Sun Exposure Map of US—This map represents the number of sunny days per year per area—lighter grays mean more sunshine, darker grays mean less sunshine.

HEALING

When I was a kid, it seems like I injured some part of my body at least once a week. There was always some bump, bruise, or cut in the process of healing. And every time I got hurt, my skin would heal quickly, without even leaving behind a scar. Sure, big injuries can have a lasting impact even on young skin, but those everyday cuts and scrapes were no big deal. Have you noticed that these days, even small cuts and scrapes seem to take a long time to get better? And when they do, sometimes there's a patch of discoloration where the injury was?

What's going on? Remember that the epidermis—the top layer of skin—is constantly growing and renewing itself. That process is part of how the skin makes repairs when you cut yourself—and like many other processes, it slows down as we age. Wounds tend to be slower to close, which can raise the risk of infection. Healing in the dermis becomes less efficient with aging, too. Healing requires special white blood cells to move in, clean the wound, and tell other cells to get to work. Skin cells have to replicate and grow, and new blood vessels have to form. All of these processes slow down as we get older.

For healthy older adults, these changes may not be a big deal. Wounds still heal, even if they do so a little more slowly. But for people who have chronic illnesses, such as problems with circulation in their legs, diabetes, or cancer, impaired or slow healing can become a serious problem. It's important to be more vigilant with cuts and bruises, especially if they seem to be taking a long time to heal. If you have a deep cut or wound, be sure to apply an antibacterial ointment and change the bandage often. If you notice that it seems to be taking an unusually long time to heal, or seems to be getting worse, see your doctor.

SPOTS

Age spots are darkened patches, like large freckles, that appear on sun-exposed areas of your skin. Age spots tend to fade if you stay out of the sun, but they don't go away completely. They're a normal part of aging.

Some people will also notice little bright red spots on their skin. These small red dots are called *cherry angiomas,* and they're made up of dilated blood vessels that didn't form correctly. You might be alarmed when you first notice a cherry angioma, but it's pretty harmless. Cherry angiomas tend to appear on the trunk of the body, but they can show up anywhere. It's pretty common for them to appear after age 40, and by the time we reach age 70, three out of four of us will have at least one. These cherry angiomas are similar to the ones that appear in infants—except that they usually disappear in the very young, and they don't disappear in the very old.

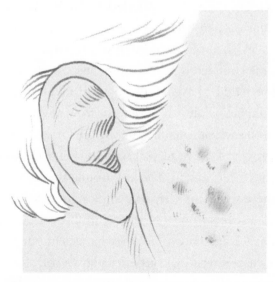

Age Spots—Also called liver spots, these dark colored marks appear on sun-exposed areas and occur due to sun damage over a number of years.

HAIR AND NAILS

Let's face it: Next to wrinkles, most people's biggest concern about the effects of aging is what happens to their hair. That includes hair loss, changes in hair texture and color, and new hair growing where you don't want it. Why does our hair change so much as we get older?

Your hair loses pigment as you age—which is a fancy way of saying, it turns gray. And it's not just the hair on your head that turns gray. By age 60, the average person has at least 50 percent gray hair on his or her body, with an even higher percentage of gray on his or her head.

The hair on our heads also tends to thin as we get older. That's because we have fewer active hair follicles as we age, and the thickness of each strand also decreases. Hair growth slows down, too. You probably noticed that you don't need to get a haircut as often as you used to once you approached middle age.

Most men are eventually affected by male pattern baldness. Twenty percent of men begin to notice some hair loss as early as puberty. By age 30, about 30 percent of men will note some baldness or become completely bald, and by age 50, nearly 50 percent of men will be bald or have a receding hairline. It's all normal.

Men can expect balding to start at the front of their hairline, with receding hair on each side making an "M" shape over their forehead. Hair at the crown of the head will start to thin, too. Eventually the balding patches meet, leaving hair just around the sides of the head.

While there's still no scientific explanation for male pattern baldness, there seems to be a hormonal link—the changes in hormone levels as we age may affect the changes in our hair follicles. But as in the case of wrinkles, genetics plays a role, too. If hair loss runs in your family, you're more likely to lose your hair. We used to think that only the genes of your maternal grandfather (your mother's father) mattered when it comes to determining your odds

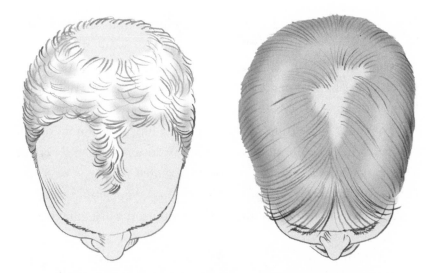

Male/Female Pattern Baldness—Men *(left)* lose hair along the forehead and on the crown of the head, while women *(right)* lose hair predominantly on the top of the head.

of losing your hair. And those genes do have a big influence. But your father's genes also play a role—if your dad was bald, chances are you will be, too. Oddly, the genes of your paternal grandfather (your father's father) don't seem to have as much of an impact. Okay . . . enough with the genetics lesson!

While it's not something many women like to talk about, there is such a thing as female pattern baldness, too. Women tend to notice it much later in life than men and typically do not lose any hair until after menopause. Women's hair usually thins all over, but female pattern baldness can also affect just the top and back of the head. Women may first notice hair loss near the part in their hair. My female patients tell me that this kind of hair loss is deeply embarrassing to them. I know it's not a lot of consolation, but it's usually a normal aspect of aging.

You can expect the hair elsewhere on your body to thin out, too, but the remaining strands often become thicker and coarser.

Look at older men and you'll probably notice bushier eyebrows and thicker hairs in the nose and ears. Older women often find themselves battling facial hair that wasn't there before. It's okay to tweeze these hairs if you want to, as long as it doesn't irritate your skin. Remember, older skin doesn't heal as well when it is irritated.

There are some times, however, when hair loss is not considered a normal part of aging. If your hair loss is sudden (over the course of a couple of months); if it's associated with pain or severe itching of the scalp; or if you feel very tired, you should see your doctor. Thyroid problems and malnutrition can cause unexpected hair loss.

Your nails won't escape aging, either. You'll find that your nails grow more slowly over time, and their appearance may change. Young, healthy fingernails and toenails are smooth, strong, and translucent. Older nails can turn dull and become more opaque, and they may take on a yellowish tint. Ridges or furrows may appear on their surfaces. Some people develop a pattern called

Skin Changes: What's Normal and Not Normal As We Age

Normal	Not Normal
Drier, rougher-looking skin	Patches of dry or scaly skin that never seem to heal
Nails that are a little yellowish and less translucent than they used to be	Whitish, yellow, or dark spots on nails
Gradual hair loss	Sudden hair loss or hair falling out in clumps
Itchy skin that improves with moisturizers	Itching all over
Age spots	New moles or lumps, or moles that change appearance

Neapolitan nails, with a line of white at the bottom, pink in the middle, and an opaque section at the fingertip. It's all normal.

When our nails turn a dark color, however, it's usually due to an infection. Whereas most other infections in our bodies are caused by bacteria, infections in our nails are caused by fungus. Fungal infections can affect your nails at any age, but they're more common as we approach middle age. A typical infection looks like whitish or blackish patches that can eventually cover the whole nail. The good news is that these types of infections rarely spread beyond the nail. The bad news is that they can be difficult to treat. They can sometimes be effectively treated with over-the-counter remedies, but your best bet is to see your doctor. You will usually need a prescription-strength antifungal medication to clear the infection.

Nails that are really thick and hard to cut, painful, brittle, bumpy, or discolored in other ways, or that peel away from the base, are not normal and should also be checked out by a doctor.

COMMON DISORDERS

As we age, it's normal to develop some skin problems. The conditions below are ones that I see commonly and am often asked about.

Dry Skin

Xerosis is the fancy medical term for very dry, scaly skin. Most adults experience this problem to at least some degree by the time they are 70 years old. It tends to be worse in climates or seasons with low humidity, but it can be a problem any time. When xerosis is particularly severe, skin can actually crack and bleed.

To battle xerosis, it's essential to keep your skin well hydrated. Look for thick creams that hold moisture in. Over-the-counter products containing urea or lactic acid are sometimes useful. Urea helps hold water in your skin; lactic acid helps smooth away the scaly, dry layer. If the air is dry where you live, a humidifier can also help.

You might hear that you should avoid taking baths or long showers if your skin is dry, but these can actually help. Bathe with a mild soap, using it sparingly. Then seal in the moisture with a hydrating skin cream as soon as you towel off. If home remedies aren't helping, check in with your doctor. Sometimes a prescription steroid cream can help soothe the skin and give it a chance to heal. Steroid creams, however, cannot be used long term, especially on the face. They can cause your skin to become thinner, and if the steroids are absorbed into your bloodstream, they may cause complications in people with diabetes or glaucoma.

Itchy Skin

Itchiness is often a direct result of dryness. Treat the dryness and the itch will go away. But as you get older, there are lots of other reasons why your skin might itch. Check your list of medications: Believe it or not, some over-the-counter painkillers can cause you to feel itchy. If the itching comes on rapidly and seems to affect you all over, it is not normal and could be a sign of a more serious illness or an allergy.

Adult Acne

It's not uncommon to see a pimple or two even when you thought you'd be long past worrying about acne. Most of the patients who come to me for acne treatment are on the younger side, but medical research tells us that getting older doesn't necessarily guarantee clear skin. In one study, trained examiners saw at least a few signs of acne in a third of adults between the ages of 45 and 58.[3] Another group of researchers asked people about their own impressions. Among the older adults, 7 percent of men and 15 percent of women said they still had acne at age 50 or above.[4] There's not a lot of data on acne in adults beyond middle age, but I wouldn't worry if an older patient told me they were continuing to see a pimple now and then.

What isn't so common, as you get older, is to have the kind of prominent acne that you see in some teens and young adults. Based on the research data, I'd expect to see this type of acne in less than 5 percent of women and maybe 1 percent of men past their mid-forties. If you're still having serious breakouts, or if you just recently started having them, see a doctor. (Actually, serious breakouts at any age would be a reason to seek treatment—we have a lot of ways to tackle acne these days.) If it's just plain old acne, you can get treatment that's tailored to older patients and therefore gentler on your skin than what would be prescribed to a teenager. Or you might find out that you actually have a different problem, like rosacea. Sometimes acnelike breakouts can also be caused by a chemical exposure at work or by a drug you're taking.

When it comes to run-of-the-mill acne, we don't know why some people still continue to break out into adulthood. Both blackheads and whiteheads develop when there is overproduction of the type of cells that line hair follicles, and a mixture of sebum and dead skin cells forms a plug. There also appears to be a link between acne and androgens: There are people whose cells don't make androgen receptors, and they don't produce sebum or develop acne. We know that androgens help regulate sebum production, and one theory is that people who have trouble with acne have sebaceous glands that are especially responsive to androgens. Other possible influences include effects of bacteria and genetics.

Sometimes older adults develop acnelike spots or bumps called *senile comedones*. (You might also hear these called solar comedones or Favre-Racouchot Syndrome.) They can look like whiteheads or blackheads, and they often show up on skin near the eyes. They're thought to be related to sun damage, with changes in the dermis allowing hair follicles to fill up with dead skin cells. Senile comedones can be removed easily by a dermatologist, although they do tend to come back over time.

Seborrheic Dermatitis

As many as a third of adults, typically between ages 30 and 65, have seborrheic dermatitis. What is it? It's a common skin condition that causes dandruff, and it can also cause flaky, scaly skin around your eyebrows, alongside your nose, around your groin, and even inside your ear canal—basically any place on the body where the glands that make sebum are especially abundant.

Seborrheic dermatitis may look bad, but it can be treated. Dandruff shampoo usually does the trick for hair. Tar and salicylic acid preparations can help in other places. Seborrheic dermatitis all over the body is not normal, however, and can indicate a more serious disease. If it persists for several weeks despite treatments, see your doctor.

Rosacea

Rosacea isn't exactly a disease of aging, but it is more common among older adults than younger ones. No one knows exactly what causes it. Rosacea involves reddening of the skin, usually on the face but sometimes involving the neck, scalp, ears, chest, or other areas of the body. It often appears in the form of red bumps that look like acne. Small blood vessels may appear as little red lines just under the surface of the skin. Rosacea can also make your nose look bulbous and bumpy.

Rosacea is nearly three times more common in women than it is in men. People with pale skin seem to be most susceptible, but anyone can develop rosacea. Lots of famous people have had rosacea, including Bill Clinton, Mariah Carey, Cameron Diaz, and William Shatner. Remember what W.C. Fields looked like? That's the classic case of rosacea.

Rosacea can be treated, so see your doctor if you notice these kinds of changes in your skin. You may be given antibiotic pills or creams, or even acne medications. Some folks may prefer laser therapy, which typically has good results.

Shingles

If you aren't already aware of a disease called shingles, odds are you'll start to hear about it as you grow older or if you care for an elderly parent. Shingles is the common name for what doctors call *herpes zoster*. That's not the same herpes virus that's transmitted via unprotected sexual intercourse. Shingles is caused by varicella-zoster virus, the same virus that causes chicken pox. If you've ever had the chicken pox—and if you're reading this book, you probably did because the chicken pox vaccine didn't exist until fairly recently—you're at risk of developing shingles. That's because the virus can linger in your body long, long after those itchy chicken pox blisters have healed. Your immune system keeps it from causing chicken pox again, but it actually can hide out in certain types of nerve cells. As you get older, your immune system can become weaker and may be less able to keep the virus from sneaking back out again.

The second time around, the varicella-zoster virus usually affects just one area or side of the body. Shingles starts with pain, itching, or burning over one section of skin. The initial symptoms usually last a

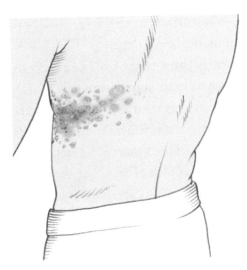

Shingles—A small constellation of painful, itchy, red bumps and blisters that occur in a narrow horizontal strand. This blistering rash only appears on one side of the body and never crosses over the midline.

few days, although sometimes they'll go on for weeks before blisters appear. Over the course of about a week, the blisters crust over and begin to heal. The classic sign is blisters on one side of the back that don't cross the center. If you see that, it's probably shingles.

You can treat the symptoms with over-the-counter pain medicines, anti-itch creams, and home remedies like cool compresses. Prescription antiviral drugs can usually speed recovery, and I recommend them. If the blisters are affecting your eyes, definitely get help immediately because your vision could be damaged.

Some people who develop shingles have lingering pain, a condition called *postherpetic neuralgia*. It tends to improve with time, but a small percentage will still have pain even a year after the blisters are gone. Treating shingles with antiviral medications can reduce the risk that the pain will linger.

You can lower your risk of getting shingles with a one-time vaccine that's recommended for adults age 60 and over. I urge my older patients to get this vaccine.

Skin Growths

I cannot tell you how many times I've been in a grocery store or at a cocktail party when someone pulls me aside and points to some type of lump or bump on their skin and asks, "Is this normal?" Everyone worries about abnormalities they see on their skin, but the dairy aisle is not the best place for dermatological consult. So I've compiled a list (below) of some of the most common skin growths that occur as we age. Hopefully, this will help put your fears to rest.

Skin tags are probably the least scary of the growths you might see. Skin tags are small, soft, fleshy growths, usually the same color as the rest of your skin. Sometimes they're attached by a short stalk. They're probably caused by the friction of skin rubbing against skin, which is why they're often found near folds on the neck and in the armpits. They're hardly ever cancerous, so the main issue is whether they bother you. If a skin tag tends to get irritated or if it just looks ugly, you can have it removed. It's usually a simple, quick procedure that can be performed right in the doctor's office. Do not try to cut these off yourself. I repeat: Do not try to cut these off yourself! Skin tags can often bleed, and I've had to treat patients who decided they could use scissors or a razor and avoid a trip to the doctor. Bad idea.

Seborrheic keratoses are dark-colored growths that look like they're "stuck on" the surface of your skin. I've even heard some doctors describe them as looking like "brown wax globs" on the skin. This tends to be a hereditary condition, and some people are especially susceptible, with 10 or more seborrheic keratoses scattered across their skin. These growths also tend to appear more often as we get older.

These growths aren't likely to become cancerous, although occasionally it can be hard to tell the difference between a seborrheic keratosis and a skin cancer; the only way to know for sure is through a biopsy. If these growths bother you, you can have them removed. Ointments and lotions don't work on these lesions, so don't waste your money on fancy products.

What many people do not realize is that these keratoses can often indicate another medical condition—the most common is diabetes. Anytime I see seborrheic keratoses on a patient, I always screen for diabetes. Make sure your doctor checks blood sugar if you or a loved one has a bunch of these "brown wax globs."

Actinic keratoses are more worrisome. These are considered precancerous. They're confined within the top layer of skin (epidermis) and aren't dangerous unless they start to grow deeper. Unfortunately, we can't be sure which ones will grow and *become* dangerous. Actinic keratoses start out as rough, scaly patches and develop into hard, rough growths. It's rare to have just one of these growths; typically, you'll have 10 or more. Even if they don't bother you, your doctor may advise you to have them removed. There are lots of ways to remove them, including minor surgery, freezing, laser treatment, and special creams that cause the growth to peel off.

Skin Cancer

Skin cancer is pretty common (it's the most common form of cancer), and it does occur in middle age and beyond. In fact, most skin cancers are diagnosed in patients over the age of 60. There seems to be a myth that skin cancer only occurs in young people. That's simply not true. Luckily, most of the skin cancers that occur in middle age and beyond can be treated pretty easily, but they need to be detected early. The most common skin cancers are:

- Basal cell carcinoma
- Squamous cell carcinoma
- Melanoma

Basal cell carcinoma is a slow-growing skin cancer that won't usually spread to other parts of the body, but it's not something to ignore. Left untreated, a basal cell carcinoma can become a large tumor. At that point, removing it becomes more difficult, and it can be disfiguring. The people at the greatest risk have fair skin that doesn't tan easily, with blond or red hair and light eyes. Sun damage raises your risk as well. Basal cell carcinomas are usually found on the head or neck, often on the nose. They can also turn up in other places, including areas that aren't usually exposed to sun.

Basal cell carcinomas can take a few different forms. They can be pinkish or whitish bumps, with a pearly appearance and prominent blood vessels. As the tumor grows, a crust forms in the center. Sometimes it will appear to heal, but it's actually still there and will continue to grow, with cycles of crusting over and healing. Basal cell carcinoma can also look like a dark growth with a pearly border; a flat, waxy-looking area; a smooth, round cyst; or a scaly spot.

Squamous cell carcinoma is less common than basal cell, and it's also more dangerous. It's a faster-growing cancer that can spread to other parts of the body, although that usually won't happen right away. Bigger, deeper tumors are more likely to spread. Again, light skin, blond hair, and blue eyes mean increased risk, but people with dark skin can get this cancer, too. Squamous cell cancers tend to turn up on sun-exposed areas like the scalp, ears, forehead, lower lip, and hands, but they can appear in other places, too. Sometimes they grow in scars or skin ulcers (open sores that extend to the dermis).

Squamous cell carcinoma tends to look like a bump or nodule that is firm to the touch. It can also look like a well-defined scaly patch, or a flat plaque on top of raised, reddened skin. Sometimes people describe it as looking like a sore that won't heal.

Melanoma is the most dangerous form of skin cancer, responsible for about 80 percent of skin cancer deaths. It's particularly deadly in the elderly. Finding a melanoma early is important, because this cancer spreads quickly once it starts growing down into the skin. Melanomas often look like an irregularly shaped freckle that seems to spread out horizontally. They're often found on parts of the body that aren't regularly exposed to the sun, so it's not clear to what degree sun exposure affects your risk.

KNOW YOUR ABC'S

Doctors use an ABCDE rule to help them decide if a spot or lump is suspicious. We typically apply this rule for melanomas, but it should be applied to any skin lump/bump you are concerned about.

- **Asymmetry.** If you draw a line down the middle, the two sides don't match. They do not look the same. A normal mole is equal on both sides and is round.

- **Border.** The edges aren't smooth; they can be bumpy or notched. Normal lesions are typically smooth to the touch.

- **Color.** The spot contains multiple shades of brown or black, or it has areas of other colors such as red or blue. A normal mole typically has one color, usually a shade of brown.

- **Diameter.** The spot or lump is wider than a pencil eraser.

- **Elevation.** The mole is raised above the surface. Most normal moles tend to be flat.

If you have a spot on your skin that meets any of these criteria, or that seems to be changing shape or is irregularly shaped, make an appointment with your doctor to have it checked out. Another important factor to keep in mind is that sores that don't heal are always considered to be abnormal. Even though I noted earlier that it takes longer for our skin to heal as we get older, a sore should still be able to heal on its own. If a sore hasn't healed for a couple of weeks, see your doctor.

FIVE TIPS TO KEEP YOUR SKIN LOOKING GOOD

1 Stay out of the sun. If you're going to be outside for long, use a good sunscreen with UVA and UVB protection and don't forget to reapply. It's also a good idea to cover up with a broad-brimmed hat, long sleeves, and long pants. (Lightweight fabrics will keep you cooler, but make sure the sun doesn't shine right through them.)

2 Moisturize. A good moisturizer will combat the dryness that comes with aging, ward off itching, and help keep your skin looking supple and smooth. And men need to moisturize, too! Ideally, you should moisturize twice a day. You might also want to consider using a moisturizer that also contains sunscreen.

3 Get checked for skin cancer. Skin cancer is linked to sun exposure, but it can also turn up on parts of your body that rarely see the sun—and that are hard for you to see, too. Have your doctor check your skin regularly for any changes. And if you see a new mole or anything else unusual, see your doctor.

4 Stay away from smoke. If you smoke, it's time to quit! If you're around people who smoke, try to get them to quit. Your lungs will thank you, and so will your skin. Smoking brings on wrinkles and makes you look old before your time.

5 Eat right. There's no magic food to keep you looking young, but eating a balanced, nutritious diet will help your whole body look, feel, and function at its best—on the inside *and* the outside.

FIGHTING AGING

If you watch late-night television, you know that there's always a "new" product out there that seems to promise eternal youth. We all know that's not possible. But there are some credible and legitimate products available that can help prevent and even undo some of the effects of aging.

Most anti-aging skin care products address the visible changes: wrinkles, age spots, and dull or dry skin. If you remember what you learned at the beginning of the chapter about the layers of your skin, you'll see why the following products can be helpful.

Before you use any kind of anti-aging product or treatment, I recommend making an appointment with a board-certified dermatologist, who can help you make a plan that's right for your skin. I also recommend caution when it comes to visiting an expert in an "anti-aging" center. I'm sure some of them are good, but my experience is that many sell products and offer recommendations that aren't based on medical fact.

Vitamin A Derivatives

Many of the anti-aging products contain some form of vitamin A, and they probably work by helping to thicken skin that has thinned with age as well as reducing the loss of collagen. Some of the ingredient names you'll see are tretinoin, retinol, retinyl acetate, retinyl propionate, retinyl palmitate, or retinaldehyde. Some of these products are available over the counter, but for others you'll need to get a prescription from your doctor. None of these elixirs will make you look 21 again, but they can make a difference. Fine lines, dark spots, pore size, and skin texture may all improve. You might eventually see changes in deeper wrinkles, too. The vitamin A–based formulas can irritate your skin, so follow the package directions carefully and stop using them if redness or irritation occurs, or if you don't notice any improvement in your skin.

Cosmeceuticals

I advise caution when it comes to cosmeceuticals. They don't have to meet the same strict standards that prescription drugs or even over-the-counter medicines must meet. This means that often, they haven't been thoroughly studied. A cosmetics company could test a product on 10 people and claim that "clinical trials have shown" that it works. From a doctor's perspective, most cosmeceuticals aren't backed by much proof. Still, some of the ingredients have shown promise and might be worth a try. Here are a few examples.

- **Alpha hydroxy acids** seem to help improve skin texture and even out skin tone. They work partly by helping to exfoliate the top layer of your skin, removing dead cells to reveal fresher-looking skin. They may also increase the production of collagen.

- **Salicylic acid** is thought to have effects similar to alpha hydroxy acids but to be less irritating to skin. This is the same ingredient in some adult acne medications.

- **Niacinamide** is a form of vitamin B_3 that's said to reduce fine lines, even out skin tone, shrink pores, and improve skin texture. Research so far suggests that over several weeks, a niacinamide-based cream might improve the look of age spots and help reduce the appearance of fine wrinkles. There's also a chance it could shrink pore size by reducing sebum production.

- **Kinetin** is a plant growth hormone. It seems that using a lotion containing kinetin could improve the texture of skin and decrease fine wrinkles. It might also help restore or maintain your skin's function as a barrier against outside irritants.

- **Vitamin C.** Research seems to suggest that vitamin C might actually work to reduce fine lines, possibly by increasing collagen production. It may also help to lighten discolored skin. The problem with using vitamin C in skin creams is that it isn't very stable and it's not very well absorbed by your skin. The companies who make these products have been working on better formulas, but right now I'm not sure you'd be getting your money's worth. Eating foods rich in vitamin C or taking supplements won't have as much of an effect.

SKIN TREATMENTS AT THE DOCTOR'S OFFICE

Over-the-counter creams and prescription drugs only go so far. If you are looking for more dramatic effects, you may consider an in-office procedure.

Microdermabrasions

Microdermabrasion uses tiny crystals to essentially sand off the epidermis, reducing wrinkles and evening out color. Lasers and chemical peels can also treat spots and wrinkles by removing a thin layer of skin. These treatments can indeed make you look somewhat younger, but they also carry a risk of scarring and discoloration.

Wrinkle-Filling Injections

Injections really can plump up skin and smooth out wrinkles, and the effect lasts for at least a few months.

Collagen has been used this way for many years, and it's sometimes used in combination with newer options. If you choose a collagen injection, you might want to consider the source of the collagen: Depending on the product, it may come from animals, from human cells grown in a lab, or even from human cadavers. It's also possible to have collagen made from a small piece of your own skin. Results usually last a few months.

There are a number of other injections that reduce wrinkles by plumping up the skin. I mentioned hyaluronic acid earlier in the chapter—remember, it holds water in the skin and helps it maintain elasticity. Depending on the product, you'll see results for a few months to a year with this type of injection.

Another filler is made from tiny spheres of calcium hydroxylapatite. This is a mineral substance found in bone, although the stuff in the injection is man-made. The idea is that it encourages the skin to make more collagen, which can mean longer-lasting results, although you might need a touch-up after a few months.

Botulinum Toxin

Botulinum toxin ("botox") shots have certainly gotten popular in recent years. Sometimes it seems there isn't a celebrity left in Hollywood who can move the muscles in his or her forehead! Botulinum toxin is the same thing that causes the symptoms of botulism, a form of food poisoning that temporarily paralyzes you. Used properly, in tiny quantities, it can weaken your facial muscles just enough that creases don't form in your skin. The idea is that if you don't make those creases, your skin won't wrinkle.

Case Study

Arnold is a 67-year-old man whose only medical problem is high cholesterol. He and his wife recently retired, and were planning an RV trip across the country. When Arnold came to see me, he was complaining of cold symptoms and wanted me to prescribe "some antibiotics to make this go away before we hit the road." I performed a quick exam, and we discussed his symptoms. I let him know that antibiotics wouldn't help relieve his cold, and offered some suggestions for managing the discomfort. But at the end of the appointment, Arnold's wife of 45 years, Cheryl, stuck her head into the exam room and asked her husband, "Did you tell him about the spot?"

Arnold looked embarrassed. "Come on, Cheryl, Dr. Whyte doesn't want to hear about that freckle."

Actually, I did. A new or changing "freckle" on a man his age could be a cause for concern. The spot his wife was referring to was on Arnold's back, so I asked him to remove his shirt. While he was undoing the buttons, he continued to apologize, saying, "I don't know what she's so worried about, I've never even gotten sunburned there."

Arnold had a number of moles on his back. Cheryl said most of them have been there "forever," but she pointed out one that she thought was new. It wasn't very big, not even as big around as a pencil eraser, but it was irregularly shaped and the color was a mix of tan and brown. I wasn't certain that it was a melanoma, but I didn't like the look of it.

Growth Hormone

Growth hormone is often advertised as an anti-aging miracle drug. It's true that your growth hormone levels decline as you age, but there's no proof that adding it back will make your skin look younger. Growth hormone can cause serious side effects, so until there's a good scientific study to support its use in fighting aging, it's not something I recommend using for anti-aging purposes.

I referred Arnold to a dermatologist so that he could get a biopsy. "Sure, doc," Arnold said, starting to put his shirt back on. "We'll stop along the way. I bet my son out in Tucson knows a good dermatologist."

Cheryl shook her head. "We're not waiting that long. Tell him, Dr. Whyte!"

I agreed. Melanoma isn't something to mess with. It's important to catch it early, because if you treat it in its earliest stages, the outlook is good. Later on, though, survival rates aren't so good. Once I explained this to Arnold, he agreed to make an appointment right away.

I also suggested that Arnold have a full screening for skin cancer, which involves a dermatologist carefully looking over your whole body to make sure there aren't any other suspicious spots. (I could do that exam for Arnold, but I think it's even better to let the dermatologist have a look.) Arnold agreed to request a full screening when he made his appointment.

A few weeks later, Arnold and Cheryl called me from the road. They kept the appointment with the dermatologist, who biopsied the "freckle" and didn't find anything else suspicious. The diagnosis? Melanoma. But Arnold was lucky. We caught it early enough that, after surgery to remove the tumor, he didn't need additional treatment. He'll need regular checkups, and he'll have to keep a careful watch for any other suspicious skin changes. Luckily, he has Cheryl to help keep an eye on him.

Treatments for Hair Loss

Here's an area where today's treatments really can fight the signs of aging. Think about how much progress we've made over the past 20 years when it comes to hair loss. When's the last time you saw someone wearing a toupee? Probably more than a decade ago.

That's because today we have more and better options. Minoxidil, which can be used by both men and women, is a medication you apply directly to your scalp, and it's available over the counter. It isn't always effective for everyone, but when it does work, it can actually stimulate new hair growth and stop hair loss from worsening. You'll get the best results if you start using it when you first notice that your hair is thinning. Despite what you might see on some commercials, you're not likely to see a full head of hair come back if you already have large bald patches. Minoxidil is a long-term commitment—if you stop using it, you'll go right back to losing your hair again.

Finasteride is another option, although it's available only for men. This prescription pill reduces levels of a form of testosterone that seems to trigger hair loss. Most men can use it without any problems, but side effects can include a decreased libido and erectile dysfunction. It can also affect blood tests used for prostate cancer screening. So be sure to let your doctor know you're taking it, if he or she doesn't already know. As with minoxidil, the effects of finasteride won't last if you stop taking it. It can also take a while to see good results—sometimes up to 2 years.

Sometimes my patients ask me if it's possible to "overdo it" with hair loss drugs. You're supposed to apply minoxidil twice a day, but will it work faster if you put some on at lunchtime, too? Would three or four times a day be even better?

Like many things in life, more isn't always better! I don't recommend using minoxidil more often than directed. One reason is because minoxidil is also used, in pill form, to lower blood pressure. If enough of it is absorbed through your skin, you could end up feeling dizzy and even putting a strain on your heart. Gaining some more hair isn't worth being dizzy all the time! If you are using minoxidil as prescribed and it isn't working for you after a few months, talk with your doctor.

Laser treatments are another popular option, though it's hard to say yet how well they work, or if there are any long-term safety concerns. There just aren't enough studies yet.

You can also look into hair replacement surgery. Basically, a hair transplant involves moving hair from the back of your head to the front, a few strands at a time. You can also have more dramatic surgery that moves a whole flap of skin around to the front of your head. "Scalp reduction" surgery removes a piece of skin from the bald spot and pulls the back and sides of your scalp closer together. If you are interested in surgery, be sure to choose your surgeon carefully. Like any surgical procedure, there are risks. These can include infections, bleeding, pain, bad reactions to anesthetics, and poor results. There have been instances of death as well even with what seems like simple surgical procedures. Also, hair replacement surgery can often be expensive. Since insurance often does not pay for procedures considered to be cosmetic.

Plastic Surgery

I can't honestly tell you if or when plastic surgery might be "right" for you as a way to combat aging. Personally, I'm not fond of the idea of having myself cut open just to look younger. Complications are rare, but they can happen, and I'm not always sure it's worth the risk. But some people do feel these procedures are worth it, and I've seen patients, friends, and colleagues who are really satisfied with the results.

I would actively recommend that a patient see a plastic surgeon for age-related changes in a few cases. For example, some people find that drooping eyelids start to impede their vision, and plastic surgery can help with that. Patients who have had significant weight loss also can benefit by having excess skin removed. Of course, if a patient is really interested in surgery to mask the signs of aging, I'll recommend that they talk with a good surgeon about what can be done.

Answers to true/false statements: False, True, False, True

Chapter 2

SHAPE AND SIZE

True or False

You will shrink an inch in height by age 60.   _____

You gain about 10 pounds a decade after age 40.   _____

Your metabolism automatically slows down
as you age.   _____

Muscle turns to fat as we get older.   _____

(Answers at end of chapter)

Have you been to a high school or college reunion lately? If you have, you probably noticed that many of your classmates look a lot different than they did 25 or 30 years ago. And I'm not just talking about how many of the men have lost their hair. Most people also seem to look a bit wider, and some even look shorter. Those members of the girls' basketball team don't seem so intimidating anymore!

Or maybe you're starting to digitize all your old photos and you find that you barely recognize the body you used to have in your twenties. Other than some wrinkles, do you feel you look the same, or has your body shape changed significantly?

I bet your body does look different today than it did 20 or 30 years ago. I know mine does. What's really happening, and why is it happening? Is getting flabby or gaining weight an inevitable part of getting older?

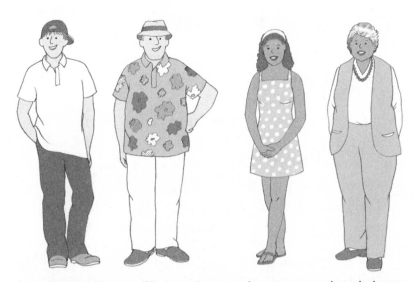

Body Shape at 18 versus 50—In our teens, we have more muscle and a lower percentage of body fat. As we age, there is a loss of lean muscle mass, which gives way to a higher percentage of body fat. This tends to gravitate toward the midsection of men and the hips, thighs, and buttocks of women.

It is true that your metabolism will likely slow down as you get older, which can contribute to an expanding waistline as the years go by. Then again, you might be surprised to learn that after about the age of 70, many people begin to *lose* weight. Either way, you don't have to sit back and accept that aging means you're never going to fit into your favorite jeans again. There's a lot you can do to keep in great shape as your body goes through the natural aging process.

In this chapter, I'll explain what we mean when we talk about metabolism and discuss how it will change as you age. Then I'll walk you through what we know about changes to fat and muscle. We'll even look at some of those "miracle" weight loss products you've probably read about or seen on TV. Sure, getting older means you might not look as great in a bathing suit as you used to, but I'll share some tips to keep your body trim, your weight stable, and your muscles strong—as well as alert you to the changes in your shape and size that are not normal.

METABOLISM BASICS

I'm sure you've heard the term *metabolism* before. When a skinny teenager wolfs down a pizza, follows it with a 20-ounce bottle of soda, and then looks around for dessert, we say, "I bet he has a fast metabolism." And we are probably right . . . sort of.

So what is metabolism? When you look at it on a molecular level, it's an extremely complicated set of processes within the body. It would take me the rest of this book to explain exactly how food gets broken down into energy, but here are a few terms you need to know to understand what is normal as we age.

Metabolic Rate

The first set of terms has to do with your metabolic rate. Metabolic rate is the amount of energy your body uses over a given amount of time. Your own personal metabolic rate changes depending on what you're doing at a particular moment: asleep or awake, sitting still or exercising, even eating versus feeling hungry. One of the biggest influences on your overall caloric needs is your *basal metabolic rate (BMR)*.

Your BMR reflects the energy needed to keep your body alive when you're doing absolutely nothing. Technically, it's how fast you're burning energy when you haven't eaten for about 12 hours, are awake and lying down, aren't moving, and aren't particularly hot or cold.

When BMR is considered across a 24-hour day, it's sometimes called *basal energy expenditure*.[1] Your BMR explains about 50 to 70 percent of your *total energy expenditure*.[2]

There's one more term that comes in handy when you're trying to understand the basics of metabolism and how it affects your size and shape. It's called *fat free mass (FFM)*. Different tissues and organs in your body burn calories at different rates, so it's important to take body composition into account. Essentially, FFM is everything in your body that isn't fat. FFM includes your bones, your muscle tissue, and the cells making up your organs—but not that spare tire around your middle or the extra jiggle in your thighs. FFM has a huge effect on your metabolic rate. Fat cells use up calories at a particularly slow rate. So when you have more fat cells than muscle cells, it makes it even more difficult to lose weight. That's one of the reasons why it's so important to keep muscle as you age.

Older adults tend to have lower BMRs than younger people. The decrease in BMR is about 1 to 3 percent per decade from age 20 to age 96, for men and women of normal weight. Again, this makes it harder to lose excess weight.

Some research suggests that the decrease in BMR as we age is the result of a loss of FFM and a relative increase in fatty tissue. "Loss of FFM" is a fancy way of saying that your muscles and other organs become smaller as you get older, so there is simply less tissue with high metabolic activity. If the ratio of fat to muscle and other organs increases, your overall metabolism appears to slow down. There is some research to suggest that in women, BMR starts falling more quickly around age 50, which could coincide with a loss of muscle and bone mass during menopause.

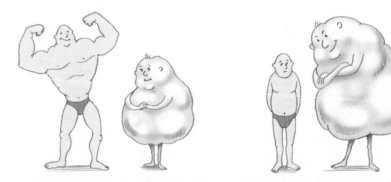

Fat-Free Mass (FFM)—Also called body composition, FFM refers to how much muscle versus fat we have. Some amount of shift of muscle to fat is normal as we age, but this can be controlled by diet and exercise.

In addition to the fall in BMR, it's also normal to see a decline in total daily energy expenditure with age. This decline probably reflects a decrease in physical activity. After all, if you're not racing to work in the morning, chasing around the kids or grandkids, or running errands throughout the day, your basal metabolic rate will decrease, and that will cause the additional pounds on the body—because we're burning fewer calories at rest. The result: weight gain. Makes sense so far?

Let's be honest: Most of us are less active and more sedentary as we age. If we get out less, exercise less, and just generally slow down, then it makes sense that we're using less energy per day. And that results in changes to our size and shape.

Changes in Muscle and Fat

Have you ever known an athlete who seemed to acquire a paunch shortly after he stopped playing football or basketball? I've noticed that people like to say, "All that muscle turned to fat." You may have heard that aging causes muscle to turn to fat, too.

Well, you've been given a lot of misinformation! Simply put, muscle doesn't "turn to fat." Take a look at the illustration on the next page showing muscle cells and fat cells under a microscope. Just like apples cannot turn into oranges, muscle cells simply can't transform into fat cells, no matter what you eat or how much time you spend in front of the TV.

There are changes that seem to go along with aging, though. Muscles do become smaller. Maybe that's why there's less flexing of the "guns" at the gym once we get past 40! And when was the last time you saw an adult stretch at the pool? The number of muscle fibers in our arm and leg muscles actually decreases as we get older. As a result, we have less strength and less endurance. So it is normal that you are not going to be able to lift five bags of groceries as easily, or walk the park as quickly, as you did 20 years ago.

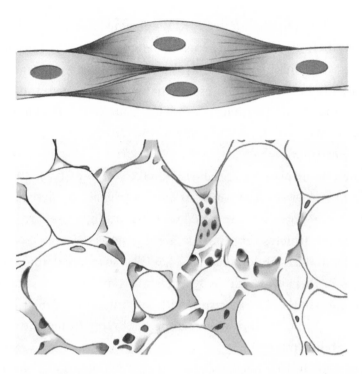

Muscle Cell and Fat Cell—Muscle cells *(top)* are tightly bound fibrous cords that stretch along the length of the muscle. Fat cells *(bottom)* are stored and packed together in globular structures that are then stored on our hips, thighs, and bellies.

Reaction time is slower, too, as is speed of movement. We simply have less flexibility than younger men and women. An important caveat to all of this is to realize that these changes are gradual over many years. If you or a loved one suddenly becomes weak, that may indicate underlying disease, and you should see your doctor.

But it's not all gloom and doom for our size and shape as we age. Getting older does not mean that you have to develop stringy muscles, flabby thighs, and jiggly arms. I'm also not saying that you should still be able to fit into those pants from 10 years ago (and I know you still have pants that old in your closet). But there is quite a bit we can do to slow down age-related changes to our bodies by staying active, watching our diets, and getting plenty of exercise.

Keeping Muscles Strong

When I first started medical school, doctors thought that aging muscles wouldn't benefit much from exercise. But we've learned a lot since then. Exercise is essential for middle-aged and older adults. Older adults might take longer than young people to see the same level of improvement, but that doesn't mean improvement won't happen.

Getting plenty of exercise won't make you look like a 20-year-old, but it does seem to ward off some of the age-related changes in body composition. Compared with older adults who are sedentary, older athletes who pursue aerobic exercise have less total body fat and less abdominal fat. They also have larger amounts of muscle in their arms and legs. Their arms and legs resist fatigue better. When they're exercising with maximal effort, their hearts even pump more blood with each beat. Staying fit tends to ward off disability, too.

Even if you don't get any exercise now, it's not too late to start. I know, sometimes the thought of exercise can be intimidating, especially if it hasn't been part of your life for a while. If you're new to exercise, recruit a friend or spouse to help you get moving. The benefits are well worth it. Resistance training, which involves using your muscles to contract against some type of external resistance, is a great way to help build strength, stability, and muscle mass to support healthy bones. Aerobic training (or "cardio") can help reduce your total body fat, give you more energy, and improve heart health. And of course, any form of exercise boosts your metabolism, which will help you to burn more calories. Studies also show that people who exercise regularly are less likely to suffer from depression, so becoming more physically active can actually help to lift your mood.

It is true that you do have to be a little more careful with your workouts as you get older. Age seems to bring less tolerance for heat and cold, and you might not be able to maintain the same level of effort during a workout that you could when you were younger. You may find that you feel out of shape sooner if you start skipping workouts, and that it's harder to get going again after a few weeks off from the gym. And please stay away from the "weekend warrior" routine, no matter what age you are. If you haven't been exercising regularly, start out slowly, get into a routine, and gradually work up to longer or more intense bouts of exercise. Don't save it all for the weekend—that's a sure recipe for injury.

Exercise Prescription

I often hear from patients and caregivers that they think they or their mothers or fathers are too frail to exercise, or that there's no real benefit if you're already over 65. That's simply not true. We tend to be overly cautious with our loved ones. You would be surprised how many elderly folks could benefit from exercise. The Centers for Disease Control (CDC) offers specific guidelines to help adults ages 65 and over stay fit.[3] Assuming one is generally healthy and in reasonably good physical shape, the CDC recommends at least:

• 2 hours and 30 minutes of aerobic exercise, of at least moderate intensity, each week. That's equivalent to about half an hour a day, 5 days a week.

• Muscle-strengthening activities at least twice a week, like weight lifting or yoga. Aim for moderate to high intensity, and be sure to work your legs, hips, back, abdomen, chest, and arms.

What do they mean by "moderate intensity"? That's exercise

that speeds up your heart rate and your breathing, although you're not so out of breath that you can't talk. If you prefer vigorous exercise—faster heart rate, harder breathing, need to catch your breath after a few words—do at least 75 minutes a week.

Remember that those are guidelines, not rules. I always tell patients that it's not about going to the gym; it's about incorporating physical activity into their everyday routines. And the key is to find activities that you enjoy, so that exercise doesn't feel like a chore. I don't know about you, but I never liked doing chores growing up. (My mother will probably tell you I never did my chores.)

Don't underestimate the value of being fit as you get older. A recent study in the *Journal of the American Medical Association* found that if you took two persons who were the same age, and had the same medical conditions, the one who was less fit was four times more likely to die within 12 years. Being fit can help you live longer and stay active for a better quality of life.

Changes in Weight

Do you know anyone who weighs the same as he or she did at 21 years old? Probably not! It's very common to gain weight as you approach and pass through your middle years. You're typically eating more, and being active less. Are you really so surprised that you're putting on pounds? After all, it's simple math:

Calories In = Calories Out

Calories In > Calories Out—> Gain Weight

Calories In < Calories Out—> Lose Weight

If you take in more calories and don't balance it by burning those excess calories, you'll gain weight. Or if you simply eat the same amount of food you always have, but you expend less energy, you'll still gain weight. And many patients have told me that they or their loved ones actually eat less, yet still are gaining weight. That can still be normal if your activity level decreases more than your food intake—meaning that if you eat only two meals a day, but you're in front of the television all day or in a recliner, the pounds are still going to add on. No doubt about it—it's much easier to put on 5 pounds than it is to lose 5 pounds as we get older.

I do want you to know, however, that many studies have found that weight tends to decline after about age 70. It's not clear exactly why. You're probably thinking, "Dr. Whyte, with all that evidence about BMR declining with age, shouldn't weight keep rising?" Great question!

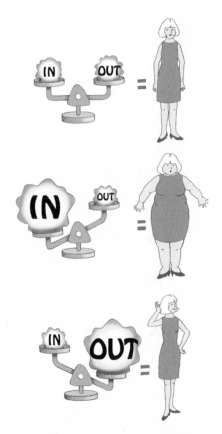

Calorie/Weight Balance—A healthy figure is a delicate balance. It is dependent on the IN—the calories you consume—and the OUT—the calories you burn with exercise and your body's natural metabolism.

One possibility is that we simply eat less as we age. In fact, there are good reasons why that may happen. Your senses of smell and taste are likely to decline with age, making food less appetizing. Changes in your digestive system may make you feel full sooner. There are even hormonal changes that can interfere with your appetite.

Body Changes: What's Normal and Not Normal As We Age

Normal	Not Normal
Decrease in height	Unintentional weight loss (> 10 lb)
Metabolism slows down	Significant muscle loss
Thinner bones	Stooped posture

But don't expect to use getting older as an automatic diet plan. In fact, significant weight loss with aging can be a sign of poor health. So if you or a loved one is unintentionally losing more than 10 pounds over a few months, it's time to get checked out.

Case Study

Jessica is a 45-year-old woman who comes in once a year for her checkup. On a recent visit, she noted that she had lost 20 pounds over the past 4 months. Normally I'd be happy to hear about such weight loss; however, Jessica was not trying to lose weight. Unintentional weight loss can indicate a serious health problem and always warrants an aggressive workup. Jessica said that she felt fine, just more tired than usual. "But I do have twin 7-year-old boys! And a puppy," Jessica explained.

I examined Jessica, drew some blood, and asked her to come back in a week. When she came back, her weight was the same, but she shared a piece of information she'd omitted on her first visit: She'd felt a lump in her armpit a month ago while doing a self breast exam. Her gynecologist had ordered a mammogram, and everything was fine.

I was concerned, so I did a more thorough exam, and I did feel a small lump in both of her armpits. Any type of lump should *always* be biopsied, so I arranged for her to see a surgeon the next day.

In this case, Jessica's biopsy came back positive for non-Hodgkin's lymphoma. Luckily, it was caught fairly early. Based on her stage, she underwent chemotherapy and is currently doing well.

Eating for Your Age

If your weight is stable, it's within a healthy range for your height, and your muscles are strong, you're probably getting the right number of calories. But as you get older, you might find that you need a little guidance to keep your weight in check.

Do you remember the old "food pyramid," with grains and breads on the bottom and junk food in that little triangle on top? These days, the food pyramid is an interactive computer program that changes according to your personal characteristics. If you go to the USDA's Web site MyPyramid.gov, you can enter your age, sex, height, weight, and activity level, and you'll get personalized information to help you determine a healthy weight.

What you'll discover, if you play around with the program a bit, is that calorie needs vary according to your age. If I enter my current age, MyPyramid.gov tells me I need 2,600 calories per day. But if I drop 20 years, MyPyramid gives me an extra 200 calories. And if I add 20 years? That's right—I get 200 fewer calories. That's without changing a thing about my height, weight, or the amount of exercise I'm getting.

Everyone is different, so you might need to eat a little more or less than the MyPyramid program tells you to. But in general, the changes that go with aging mean that after about age 40, you'll probably need fewer calories than you did when you were younger.

STANDING TALL

Remember when you stood next to your grandmother as a kid, and you and she were practically the same height? She'd probably make a joke about having shrunk—but she was right. Starting around age 40, height declines by about half an inch per decade. After age 60, it can decline even faster. Part of this is probably just a fact of life. It's not your imagination that those pants seem longer or that miniskirt now extends to your knees! Your spine is made of bony vertebrae with cushions, called disks, in between. As you age, those disks get compressed and the curve of your spine changes.

There's another reason why some older adults lose height, though, and that's osteoporosis. *Osteoporosis* is a medical term for thinning of the bones. Normally, your bones are at their toughest when you're in your mid to late twenties. By the time you're in your forties, you've begun to lose bone mass. The loss of bone mass is particularly pronounced in women after menopause, but it

FOUR TIPS TO MAINTAIN NORMAL SHAPE AND SIZE AS YOU AGE

1 Eat at least one whole fruit and vegetable a day. I know, I know . . . dietary guidelines say to eat more. I find patients get so confused by all the different recommendations and what counts as a serving that they end up eating no fruits and vegetables. Make it a point to have at least one of each every day. More is even better.

2 Weigh yourself weekly. Everyone has an estimate of how much they weigh, but guess what? It's usually wrong. I wish my patients weighed only as much as they think they do, but unfortunately most of them underestimate their weight by 10 or more pounds. Studies show that people who weigh themselves once a week are more likely to maintain a healthy weight.

3 Do resistance training at least twice a week. As I mentioned earlier, cardio is not enough as you get older. You have to either lift weights or use your own body weight to keep muscle mass and prevent bone loss. If you do only one exercise, make it a pushup. But do 50 to 100 of them!

4 Get a checkup every year, and ask your doctor to check your blood sugar level, kidney function, and your lipids (total cholesterol, HDL, LDL, and triglycerides).

happens in men as well. The picture below illustrates loss of bone mass. Inside normal bones is a sort of latticework structure with small, relatively uniform holes. As you lose bone mass, the lattice gets weaker and the holes get bigger. When you have osteoporosis, the inside of your bones looks sort of like Swiss cheese.

This thinned, osteoporotic bone is easily broken. Someone with osteoporosis can break a rib just by coughing too hard. In your spine, weakened vertebrae can collapse on themselves, stealing away your height. Fractured vertebrae can also change the shape of your spine, leading to stooped posture with a noticeable "hump."

Once you notice the first signs of osteoporosis, it's nearly impossible to reverse the disease. The key is to work on preventing further damage, and to prevent the condition in the first place. You can reduce your risk of osteoporosis by getting regular exercise, plenty of calcium, and a generous amount of vitamin D. Weight-bearing exercise, which requires your body to work against gravity, is your best bet to build bones. Weight-bearing exercises include walking, running, playing tennis, and even dancing. If you or a loved one

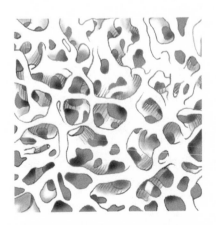 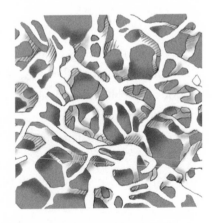

Normal versus Osteoporotic Bone—Healthy bone *(left)* is densely packed with plenty of supporting strands. Bone affected by osteoporosis *(right)* loses its dense structure, with fewer reinforcing fibers.

already has osteoporosis, or think you might, you will need to check with your doctor before you start an exercise program.

MAGIC PILLS

Patients are always asking me if there's a magic pill out there to give them back the body they had in high school or college. Let's look at some of the most common products I'm asked about.

Growth Hormone

Back in 1990, there was an article in the *New England Journal of Medicine* that seemed to draw the conclusion that growth hormone could reverse the effects of aging. The *New England Journal of Medicine* is a prestigious medical journal, and many people jumped on the idea of growth hormone as a fountain of youth. You can now buy all kinds of products that claim to make you younger, from expensive prescription growth hormone shots to over-the-counter pills that supposedly stimulate growth hormone production.

But does it work?

Growth hormone is naturally produced by the pituitary gland, a small gland that sits at the base of the brain. Children need growth hormone to develop properly and reach their full height. If you have pituitary disease, you could experience growth hormone deficiency as an adult, leading to low energy, increased body fat and decreased lean body mass, heart problems, and insulin resistance. Some of these things sound quite similar to the changes that can accompany aging, don't they?

In fact, as you get older, secretion of growth hormone naturally declines. It makes sense, then, that researchers have wondered if adding back some growth hormone might reverse the changes of aging. Well, what seems to make sense doesn't always actually make sense.

Although growth hormone may increase the size of muscles, it doesn't seem to increase their strength or improve their function. And strength training plus growth hormone doesn't seem to offer any more benefit than strength training alone.

The risks of growth hormone can be quite serious. It can make your heart grow abnormally large as well as cause damage to your liver and thyroid gland.

It's possible that future studies will teach us more about growth hormone, and maybe someday we'll understand more about its relationship to aging. For now, unless you have a disease such as a pituitary tumor that causes a true growth hormone deficiency, don't mess with it.

DHEA

Dehydroepiandrosterone (DHEA) is another substance being touted as a solution to aging. It's made by the adrenal glands, which sit just above your kidneys. Its full role in the body is unknown, but we do know that it's transformed into androgens and estrogens within other tissues. Like growth hormone, the amount of DHEA in your body declines with age.

In rats and mice, giving supplemental DHEA can prevent obesity, diabetes, cancer, and heart disease. But rats and mice don't make DHEA the way humans do, so it's hard to say if these studies mean anything unless you are a mouse or a rat. In humans, there are several small and preliminary trials to suggest benefits from DHEA on a range of age-related changes. The problem is that not all studies have found the same results, and some contradict one another. Right now, we really can't say what taking DHEA supplements might—or might not—do for you. And even more importantly, we don't know if it might do any harm. So it's probably best to wait until we have more information that benefits outweigh risks.

Answers to true/false statements: True, False, True, False

Chapter 3

EATING, BURPING, AND . . .

True or False

Most people become constipated as they get older. _____

Diarrhea should always be evaluated by a doctor. _____

You should have a bowel movement at least
three times a week. _____

We do not need to eat as much as we get older. _____

(Answers at end of chapter)

We seem to start making lots of noises as we get older, don't we? I'm talking noise from our mouths, stomachs, and "the other end" too. Burping, belching, farting, rumbling . . . It is all normal—to a point.

As we approach middle age and beyond, digestion does slow down. Depending upon exactly what is going on, our bodies are going to make some noises as food moves through them. To understand what is normal and what is not normal, let's review the digestive process.

DIGESTION

Do you remember learning about digestion in your middle school health class? The teacher probably told you to think of your digestive system as a food processor. That's pretty basic—and mostly true.

The digestive system is essentially one large tube that breaks down food. And it is a pretty large tube—more than 30 feet if you stretched it out end to end!

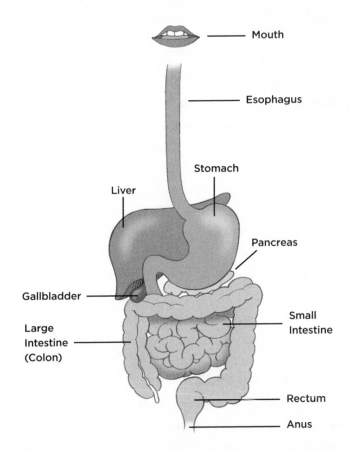

Digestive System—Everything from our teeth and tongue to our rectum and anus are included. These organs all work hard to break down the food we eat and turn it into nutrients and energy.

Let's start at the top—literally. Digestion begins in the mouth. Our saliva contains enzymes that help to break down the molecular structure of food, making it easier for the rest of the body to digest.

From there, food particles move down the esophagus into the stomach and then to the small intestine; they're then off to the large intestine, and finally the food particles are expelled from the rectum through the anus. Along the way, organs such as the liver, the gallbladder, and the pancreas get into the act, helping with digestion.

Each organ plays a different role, so there's potential breakdown in the process at every step. And truthfully, aging can cause some problems along the way. For instance, let's go back to the top. One of the parts of our bodies that we often overlook when we are young is our teeth. Most of us just don't care for them as well as we should. As a result, folks sometimes lose teeth to decay and cavities, or the remaining ones are not as strong as they used to be. Many people also suffer from gum disease. (You probably don't floss—but you should!) All of these problems can make it more difficult to chew food, which means that the food isn't broken down effectively for the other parts of the digestive process.

It is through contractions that food is propelled down into the stomach. Most people don't realize that the esophagus is actually made of muscle. As we approach middle age and beyond, the muscles get weaker, thereby making it more difficult to swallow. You might have an elderly parent who has suffered a stroke, and now has difficulty swallowing food. That's because a stroke impacts your muscles, including the esophagus. The contractions are also not as powerful, so food moves more slowly through the esophagus. That can result in food particles getting stuck.

I bet you didn't realize there is a special type of sphincter, or valve, between the esophagus and the stomach. That's important to understand because when the valve doesn't work well, acid from the stomach can shoot back up into the esophagus. This causes us to then experience burning—we call it reflux or heartburn. As we approach middle age, that sphincter doesn't always work as well as it used to.

As we get older, the stomach decreases its production of digestive enzymes. As a result, food may not be digested as well as it should be. Sometimes people will have decreased production of vitamins, including vitamin B_{12}—low levels of this vitamin can lead to anemia, which we sometimes see in the elderly.

All of these changes can make it more difficult to get the nutrients we need, in the proper amounts. In addition, we might eat less due to some of these changes as well as our decreased metabolism. So it is especially important to be aware of what we include and don't include in our diets as we get older. Supplementing with vitamins is often necessary.

So let's go back to understanding why we're making noises . . .

Belching

I'll cut to the chase—burping is caused by swallowing air. Don't we normally do that? Actually, we don't. Air is supposed to go down the windpipe (trachea), not down the esophagus into the stomach. So belching is not normal, although it is not serious.

We do it more often as we age because we might have dentures that don't fit properly, or we may not chew our food as well as we used to. Some other causes include drinking carbonated beverages quickly, and even chewing gum. It might be embarrassing, but it's harmless.

Got Gas?

In medicine, we call it flatulence. What's the cause? Gas is created through the breakdown of bacteria in our intestines and expelled through our rectums. Some bacteria release a gas when being digested. It's actually normal. The gases are harmless. I know, you've probably seen a video on YouTube where someone (usually a bored teenager) puts a match by his rectum and "lights" his gas. Guess what? That simply doesn't happen in real life. If you're passing gas, you're not going to create a fire!

Most of the time, gas doesn't have an odor. When there is an odor, it's usually related to food intake. As you probably know, some of the main culprits are baked beans, oats, corn, cabbage, and cauliflower. If you are lactose intolerant and you eat dairy foods, you might expel gas.

Below are some other symptoms and conditions that I get a lot of questions about every week.

Constipation

We all get constipated, don't we? It's pretty common, affecting more than 50 million people a year. As we get older, it's even more common. And if you're a woman or a man over 65, you're more likely to become constipated.

What do I mean by constipation? After all, do we know how many bowel movements a day or week is normal? Actually, we do. Constipation is defined as having a bowel movement fewer than three times per week. In addition, stools from constipation are typically dry, small, hard, and cause pain when being eliminated. You might have to strain to get the stool out. As a result, people sometimes become "backed up" and develop bloating or fullness, which can result in belly pain.

I must tell you—half of the people who tell me they are constipated actually are not. Some people think they are constipated if they do not have a bowel movement every day. However, you don't need to have a daily bowel movement. The number of bowel movements you have is determined by how much you eat, what you eat, and how active you are. As long as you're making a bowel movement three or four times a week, you're fine.

To understand constipation, it helps to know how the colon, or large intestine, works. As food moves through the colon, the colon absorbs water from the food while it forms waste, which is our stool. Muscle contractions in the colon then push the stool toward the rectum. By the time stool reaches the rectum, it should be solid, because most of the water has been absorbed.

Constipation occurs when the colon absorbs too much water or if the colon's muscle contractions are slow. That results in the stool moving too slowly through the intestines. As a result, stools can become hard and dry. Some common causes of constipation are poor nutrition (specifically lack of fiber), lack of physical activity, and dehydration. And our medications can be a source of constipation, too. It's not that common, but some diuretics as well as blood pressure medications, specifically calcium channel blockers, can make us constipated. Pain medications, specifically narcotics, can make our bowel movements less frequent. Iron supplements are another cause of constipation, but if you take iron, you probably already know that (those pills are pretty big, aren't they?).

What's the Real Story on Fiber?

Constipation is almost always temporary and can be relieved through diet and lifestyle choices. People who eat a high-fiber diet are less likely to become constipated. A diet with enough fiber (20 to

35 grams each day) helps the body form normal—soft but bulky—stool. High-fiber foods include beans, whole grains and bran cereals, fresh fruits, and vegetables. I understand that for some people it's hard to consume enough fiber. I remember my grandfather mixing the orange Metamucil in water at night—"Keeps me regular," he used to say. He was right. If necessary, you can take a fiber supplement such as Metamucil or Fiberall. Nowadays, they also come as tablets, wafers, and pills. It's important that you always take a fiber supplement with water.

Speaking of water, it does help to increase your fluid intake if you feel yourself becoming constipated. The extra liquids will usually make the stool a little softer, making it easier to expel.

It also helps to be active. Regular exercise actually helps your bowels to make normal stool.

Most people who are constipated do *not* need laxatives. If you need one in the short term, I usually recommend Dulcolax, milk of magnesia, or Miralax. But do not use a laxative for more than 2 days. I've actually seen people become addicted to laxatives—and that is a very bad thing.

If constipation continues off and on for 3 months, it is definitely not normal; you should see your doctor, who will typically perform a colonoscopy or barium enema x-ray.

Diarrhea

Now let's move to the opposite of constipation—diarrhea.

Diarrhea is loose, watery, and frequent stool. By definition, a person with diarrhea typically passes stool more than three times a day. The volume of stool and water can be sizable—it can be more than a quart of stool a day. Along with watery stool, we often experience cramping and bloating. Nausea sometimes is present, depending on the cause of the diarrhea.

Most diarrhea is acute, lasting only a couple of days. Having acute diarrhea is normal—and it happens at every age. The average adult has about four or five episodes every year. Diarrhea is usually mild and goes away quickly without complications.

Diarrhea is considered chronic when you have had loose or frequent stools for more than 4 weeks—that is not normal. Just because we approach middle age and beyond does not mean we should develop chronic diarrhea.

What's happening to cause diarrhea? Basically, our waste products are moving too quickly through the intestines and out through the rectum; stool has not had time to form properly. Stomach flu (the medical term is viral gastroenteritis) is the most common cause of diarrhea. Other causes can include food poisoning and medications. Medications—especially antibiotics but also blood pressure medications, cancer drugs, and antacids containing magnesium—are often overlooked as a cause of diarrhea. Numerous medical conditions can also cause diarrhea; typical ones are Crohn's disease, ulcerative colitis, celiac disease, irritable bowel syndrome, and diabetes. If you are lactose intolerant and drink milk or eat cheese, you likely will get diarrhea—but you probably already know that.

In general, diarrhea clears up on its own. However, I do get more concerned about diarrhea than I do about constipation. That's because diarrhea can cause you to become dehydrated fairly quickly. Typically, when we have diarrhea, we don't eat or drink anything. Dehydration is particularly dangerous as we get older. Left untreated, it can quickly lead to problems that will exacerbate preexisting health conditions. Here's a useful tip: Although water is extremely important in preventing dehydration, it does not contain the electrolytes the body needs when it's battling diarrhea. I recommend you try to drink fruit juices and sports drinks as well as soups. Most of them contain sodium, potassium, and other electrolytes your body needs to function well; they also replace the ones being lost in the watery stool. I've seen numerous elderly folks who became dehydrated after several days of diarrhea. If you have heart problems, losing potassium can be life threatening.

Diarrhea is particularly dangerous and typically not considered normal if you have any of the following:

- Intense, chronic abdominal pain
- Fever of 102° F or higher
- Blood in stools—it could appear red, black, or tarry

Case Study

Kerrianne is 50 years old. She is in pretty good health; she stays fairly active and watches what she eats. She works full-time at a day care center. "The kids are so cute," she always tells me. Kerrianne recently called the office to tell me that for the past 2 days, she's been having watery stools. "I think it's probably from the kids, but I wanted to make sure I don't need an antibiotic," she commented. I asked her about fever—she didn't have one. I asked if she noticed blood in the stools; she said no. I asked her if she had any belly pain, and she said, "Just a few cramps." I told her it was probably just a virus, and she should rest and drink plenty of fluids. "Understood," Kerrianne noted.

Two days later I got a call from the local Emergency Room saying that Kerrianne was being admitted for dehydration. I went to the hospital to check on her and ask what had happened. "I know I was supposed to drink fluids, but I started to feel lousy," she said. "I couldn't keep anything down, and water was making me bloated. It didn't seem at the time to be that serious. I thought I could just ride it out."

Luckily, Kerrianne had a baseline of good health. She spent the night in the hospital and was administered IV fluids until she was rehydrated. She made a full recovery, but her story serves as a cautionary tale. It's very important to drink fluids when you have a bout of diarrhea.

If you experience any of these, there's usually a more serious problem.

In most cases of diarrhea, replacing lost fluid to prevent dehydration is the only treatment necessary. Just like with constipation, I do not usually recommend medicines to stop diarrhea. Antibiotics may help only if the diarrhea is from a bacterial infection. If the diarrhea is from a viral infection, we definitely do not want to stop it since that is the body's method to get rid of the toxin. I know diarrhea isn't comfortable for many folks, but in most cases it's totally normal.

COLON CANCER

Do you remember when Katie Couric underwent a colonoscopy on live television? I'm grateful to Katie for raising awareness of a cancer that strikes people in middle age and beyond. Unfortunately, many of my patients don't remember Katie talking about colon cancer, and I'm concerned we are not doing as much as we can to screen for and prevent it. It is the third most commonly diagnosed cancer and the second highest cause of cancer deaths, so we need to take action now.

Colon cancer is cancer of the large intestine. Most colon cancers begin as small, noncancerous clumps of tissue, called polyps. As a result, if we diagnose it early, people can often be cured—unlike some other cancers.

There are several risk factors that you should know that predispose you to developing colon cancer. These include:

- Age older than 50
- African American
- History of colon polyps
- Obesity
- Diet high in red meat

- Ulcerative colitis and Crohn's disease
- Family history of colon cancer
- History of ovarian or breast cancer
- Smoking
- Heavy use of alcohol

Symptoms of colon cancer can include:

- Blood in the stools
- Unintentional weight loss
- Change in bowel habits—either lots of diarrhea or frequent constipation
- Persistent belly discomfort

Most of the time, however, there are no symptoms. That's why screening is so important.

So who needs to be screened and when? The general rule is that screening should start at age 50 unless you are at higher risk, such as having a family history of the disease. Doctors chose age 50 since more than 90 percent of colon cancer is diagnosed in people older than 50. If you're at higher risk, you may need to start at age 40 or sooner.

There are several screening tests for colon cancer. The best one, and the one that most people seem most fearful of, is the

Gastrointestinal Health: What's Normal and Not Normal As We Age	
Normal	**Not Normal**
Bowel movement at least every 3 days	One bowel movement every 4 days
Diarrhea for 2 days	Diarrhea for 3 days or more
Stomach pain for less than a day	Persistent abdominal pain
Brown stools	Blood in the stool (dark stools or floating stools)

colonoscopy. This involves inserting a long, thin, flexible tube with a tiny video camera attached to the end into the rectum. This allows the doctor to look at the entire colon, which is important so that any suspicious spots or growths can be biopsied or removed.

Other screening tests can include a CT scan, special x-rays called barium enemas, or some stool tests that look for DNA markers. Again, I think the best one is the colonoscopy. The good news is that since colon cancer grows slowly, if your colonoscopy results are normal, you won't need to do it again for 10 years.

What can you do to prevent colon cancer? Eat a diet rich in fruits, vegetables, and whole grains; reduce consumption of red meat to two or three times a week; and drink alcohol only in moderation—by moderation, I mean no more than two drinks a day. Don't smoke. Be active; engage in exercise for 30 minutes, 3 or 4 days a week. Some studies also suggest a link between taking aspirin once a day and decreased risk of colon cancer. A daily aspirin regimen does carry its risks, though, so be sure to discuss it with your doctor.

"I THINK I HAVE AN ULCER"

I bet you or someone you know has had an ulcer at some point. After all, our lives have become very stressful. How many times have you or a friend said, "This job is going to give me an ulcer"?

Peptic ulcer disease (PUD)—the medical term for ulcers in the stomach or duodenum (the first part of the small intestine)—is a very common condition, affecting nearly one out of eight adults. Basically, it's a sore in the lining of the stomach or duodenum. Just like you can get a sore on your skin, you can get a sore in the lining of your stomach.

What causes a sore to develop there? The stomach produces acid to break down food. To prevent the acid from burning through the stomach, it's lined with a thick protective layer that has a coating of mucus.

If the protective layer is damaged, we become more prone to developing an ulcer. The most common causes of ulcers are infections and use of nonsteroidal anti-inflammatory drugs (NSAIDs).

Would you believe that a bacterial infection in the stomach actually can cause an ulcer? We learned that only about 20 years ago! The bacteria *Helicobacter pylori* (*H. pylori* for short) is one of the most common bacterial infections in the world. When it gets into the stomach, it can damage the protective layer, thus causing an ulcer to develop.

Typical NSAIDs include aspirin, ibuprofen, and naproxen. That doesn't mean that you will always develop an ulcer if you take NSAIDs; NSAIDs can be very helpful in pain relief. But if you take NSAIDs regularly, you may be predisposed to developing an ulcer, so be cautious if you feel any symptoms.

How do you know if you might have an ulcer? Ulcers can cause gnawing, burning pain in the upper abdomen. These symptoms frequently occur following a meal and can last for several hours. The burning sensation can also occur during the night; many patients tell me they cannot sleep because it's so intense. Still others say they are always hungry or that food feels like it is getting stuck in their throats. Black stools may also occur. None of these symptoms are normal.

If you've been taking Tums or borrowing someone's Zantac for relief from these symptoms, you probably have an ulcer. The only way to find out for sure is to go to your doctor. We base the diagnosis on symptoms, a blood test and/or breath test, and sometimes even endoscopy (putting a tube with a light down your throat and into your stomach to see what's going on).

Treatment of ulcers is pretty straightforward. If your doctor determines that the ulcer was caused by a bacterial infection, he or she will usually prescribe a 2-week course of antibiotics and a proton pump inhibitor. These are medications that reduce acid production. You probably have heard of them; examples include Prevacid, Prilosec, Protonix, and Nexium. If the ulcer developed as a result of NSAIDs, your doctor will probably just suggest that you switch to a different type of pain medication.

WHERE'S MY GALLBLADDER?

The gallbladder is a sac located right under the liver. It stores and concentrates the bile that is produced in the liver. Bile is important since it helps digest fat. When we eat a fatty meal, the gallbladder releases bile into the small intestine, and it starts chewing up fat. That's how it is supposed to work normally.

Gallbladder disease includes inflammation, infection, and stones. You probably know someone who has had their gallbladder removed or who has had gallstones. Gallstones are small,

FIVE TIPS FOR GI HEALTH

1 As you get older, it's especially important to be aware of your nutrient intake. You're more prone to becoming malnourished, especially if you eat less due to gastrointestinal discomfort. Talk with your doctor about adding nutritional supplements or vitamins to your daily regimen, especially if you've cut out entire food groups from your diet.

2 Aim to get 20 to 35 grams of fiber a day from a variety of food sources. If you have trouble eating high-fiber foods, consider taking a fiber supplement.

3 Don't smoke. (Do I really need to explain why . . . again?!)

4 Get screened for colon cancer at age 50 unless you have a family history (then start at age 40 or earlier).

5 Stay hydrated. You might not need eight glasses of water a day, but at least aim for four.

pebble-size masses that form when the bile stored in the gallbladder hardens. Gallbladder disease affects about 20 percent of women (women usually develop the disease in their forties) and 10 percent of men (men usually develop the disease in their fifties).

You can have gallstones without any symptoms—indeed, many folks have gallstones and don't even realize it because the stones never cause any problems. It is only when the stones become large enough that they block the bile duct in the gallbladder, causing pressure and discomfort, that most people become aware of having stones. As you can imagine, blocked ducts are not normal. Bile backs up, and it can cause yellowing of the skin and eyes (jaundice). The blockage also causes pain that is typically felt in the right upper quadrant of the abdomen. This pain may be accompanied by nausea and vomiting as well. Usually the stones don't completely block off the duct, so the pain comes and goes—almost always after a fatty meal because that's when the bile is being released.

If you think you may have a gallstone, see your doctor. He or she will probably do ultrasound to determine if your gallbladder is functioning normally. If it is not, or if your gallbladder is continually causing you pain, your doctor may suggest surgery to remove it. There are no known health risks associated with living without a gallbladder. Today, most gallbladder surgeries are minimally invasive with the use of a laparoscope. Other treatment options include using ultrasound to smash the stones, or administering a drug to dissolve them, although that's often a slow process. Gallstones are more common if you are overweight, have diabetes, are taking cholesterol-lowering drugs, or if you are female or of Native American or Mexican American descent. You can help prevent gallstones by maintaining a healthy weight and eating a healthy, fiber-rich diet.

Answers to true/false statements: False, False, True, True

KEEPING CONTROL

It's one of the most common and embarrassing problems for many
of us as we get older—keeping control of our urine output. Other
than sex, it seems like urination is the topic most people don't
want to talk about. (If you've been watching reality television, I
know folks out there talk all the time about both of those things,
but that's just not normal!)

As we age, it's normal to have some problems urinating. But
those problems are probably not what you think. Because few people talk about it even with their doctors, many people do not realize what is normal and what is not normal.

WHAT'S WHAT?

To start off, let's begin with definitions.

When you leak urine when you don't want to, it's called urinary incontinence. Essentially, you didn't mean to pee and you simply couldn't control it.

There are basically three types of urinary incontinence:

1. **Stress incontinence.** Any effort or exertion, such as sneezing, laughing, coughing, or exercising, causes urine to leak. Perhaps you attended a comedy club and had a small "accident" while being entertained; or while coughing from a cold, you noted your underwear was wet. This type of incontinence is the most common kind of urinary problem in younger women; it's also the second most common type of incontinence in older women. It may also occur in older men after prostate surgery. In fact, up to a third of men who have had surgery on their prostates experience stress incontinence.

2. **Urge incontinence.** Leakage of urine is accompanied by or preceded by urgency. This is when you have difficulty holding in your urine until you reach the bathroom. You have an urge to urinate and worry that you're not going to make it to a toilet in time. Patients often will say that they feel an urge to urinate after drinking even a small amount of water. This is also the type of incontinence that occurs for some people when they hear running water. I know some people will turn on the water when they need to urinate, but that's actually not a normal thing to do.

3. **Mixed.** This type includes components of both stress and urge incontinence.

There's also something called *overactive bladder.* You may have seen some television commercials that talk about the "got to go" feeling. Overactive bladder involves urinary frequency and urgency with or without urge incontinence.

"Hesitancy" describes difficulty in initiating urination, resulting in a delay in the onset of voiding after you feel ready to pass urine.

Do you or your spouse regularly awake in the middle of the night with an urge to use the bathroom? The urge to urinate in the middle of the night is called *nocturia,* and it's not a normal part of aging. The normal pattern of urination is a decrease in urine output at night.

Occasional nocturia is common in nearly half of men and women once they reach age 50. What do I mean by occasional? Less than once a week. When comparing men and women, up to age 60, more women than men have nocturia; the sex ratio reverses after 60 years of age with more men than women getting up at night to go to the bathroom. And with each decade over 60, more people do it, so it can be common. But regardless of age or gender, you should not be getting up more than twice a night to relieve your bladder. Any more often than twice a night is not normal and requires a trip to the doctor's office.

Like the different types of incontinence, getting up at night to urinate can indicate more serious disease(s) such as diabetes, congestive heart failure, kidney disease, sleep apnea, or even Parkinson's. Don't dismiss it as a normal part of aging.

It's important to distinguish nocturia from bed-wetting (known as enuresis) since they have different causes. Bed-wetting in adults is rare—fewer than 5 percent of adults are affected. Adults who experience bed-wetting should always be seen by a urologist. Causes are numerous and can include neurological disorders, anatomical abnormalities, cancer, and anxiety disorders.

HOW URINE IS MADE

Why does getting older make us have problems "going to the bathroom"? Well, the ability to make urine is influenced by several factors. Think of it as an elaborate plumbing system. The urinary system needs to be structurally intact; we also need to have good neurological control of the system, and that requires us to have good mental function. We also need to be mobile to get to the toilet, and we need to have finger and hand dexterity to loosen our clothing garments.

The process of making urine is pretty fascinating. It is the body's process of removing harmful waste, such as urea, the waste from foods that contain proteins (like meats, poultry, and vegetables) that have been broken down by the body. The kidneys' job is

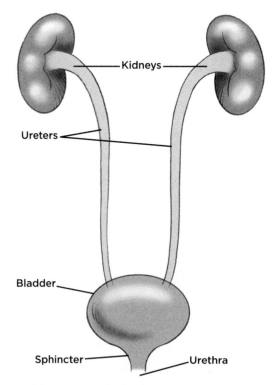

Urinary System—This system works hard to produce, store, and eliminate urine.

to then filter urea from the bloodstream. While traveling through the kidneys, the urea, water, and other waste combine to form urine. Urine then travels through two tubes called the ureters to the bladder. The bladder is the final stop for urine before you seek the bathroom to urinate. When the bladder becomes full and it starts to stretch, a nerve tells the brain it's time to urinate. (Actually, the bladder starts to send a signal to urinate when it is half-full, but the brain waits to send the signal to urinate until we consciously want to do so.)

You've probably seen those survivor shows (perhaps on Discovery Channel) or heard reports about hikers drinking their own urine when stranded in the desert without water. Urine is indeed sterile (free of bacteria)—to a point. When you pee, urine can be contaminated by bacteria on your skin. So when you're out hiking, bring enough water and you won't have to worry about whether your urine is sterile.

You might be surprised to learn that the capacity of the bladder is only 1 to 2 cups. That's not a lot of space, and it's important to keep in mind when you are having urinary problems.

Getting older does work against us in terms of maintaining normal bladder function. Increased age is associated with decreased bladder capacity (remember it's only 1 to 2 cups normally) and decreased bladder function. So as we get older, those factors impact our ability to make, hold, and control urine.

If I asked a group of people what they considered to be a normal number of times to go to the bathroom a day, most would have no clue. Some people can't even estimate how many times a day they urinate. Well, the answer is seven. Seven is the magic number—meaning it is normal to urinate up to seven times a day. It's generally abnormal to urinate eight or more times a day.

There are some warning signs that you should be aware of that require prompt attention by a medical professional. These include anytime you see blood in your urine or anytime you have trouble urinating while at the same time you are experiencing pain in your belly, groin, or pelvic area.

WHO'S MOST AFFECTED?

Urinary problems are usually thought of as a condition affecting women. That's mostly true, and in general, twice as many women as men are affected. This is partly due to the female anatomy as well as the impact pregnancies have on the urinary system. However, you'll be surprised to learn that for some urination problems, that ratio changes as we approach middle age and beyond.

Men also have problems urinating, and these problems can occur throughout their lifetimes. The problems increase as men age. Typically, most men don't begin to notice problems until around age 60. But by that age, about 20 percent of men experience problems with urinating. By the age of 85, nearly 35 percent experience difficulty urinating. This is not surprising since the majority of urination problems experienced by men are related to *benign prostatic hypertrophy* or *benign prostatic hyperplasia (BPH)*.

If you're a male and you're over 60, you probably have heard of BPH. In simple terms, BPH means the prostate is enlarged—the prostate gets larger as we get older due to the prolonged period of time it's been exposed to male hormones. The enlarged prostate causes problems with urination because eventually the prostate gets big enough to stop the outflow of urine from the bladder (specifically the urethra). Symptoms typically include trouble starting/stopping urination, increased frequency, and getting up at night to urinate. Symptoms of BPH can be the same as those for prostate cancer, so if you are having these symptoms, you should definitely see your doctor for a prostate exam and a prostate-specific antigen (PSA).

Bladder Control: What's Normal and Not Normal As We Age

Normal	Not Normal
Getting up twice a night to pee	Getting up three times or more a night to pee
Urinating up to seven times a day	Urinating more than eight times a day
Urine that is clear to light yellow in color	Dark urine or blood
One or two urinary tract infections a year	Monthly urinary tract infections

QUESTIONS TO ASK AND/OR ANSWER

Even though urinary problems are more common than most people think, no one wants to admit that he or she has a problem with bladder control. So here are the questions I ask patients to determine if bladder control is normal.

- Do you have or have you ever had loss of urinary control?
- Do you ever leak or lose urine when you cough, laugh, or sneeze?
- How often do you have difficulty holding your urine until you can get to the bathroom?
- Do you ever use pads, tissue, or cloth in your underwear to catch urine?

If you answer yes to any of these questions, you need more tests.

There are certain factors that put you at increased risk for urinary problems. If you or an elderly loved one has any of the following, you're more likely to develop incontinence: high blood pressure, obesity, BPH, prostate cancer, diabetes, dementia, stroke, and heart disease.

You might be surprised to learn that prescription medications sometimes can cause problems with urination; the most likely culprits are diuretics and antidepressants. I'm always a little surprised that people sometimes forget that their diuretic—a medication that makes them lose water by urination—may actually be causing their urination problems. We sometimes overlook the obvious!

I had a patient, Bessie, a while back who used to tell me, "Doctor Whyte, I am what I ate." This statement holds true especially

FOUR TIPS TO MAINTAIN A HEALTHY URINARY SYSTEM

1 Decrease fluid intake at bedtime. I know some friends who like to keep a glass of water on their nightstand; my wife actually does that. But if you're getting up at night to urinate, it might be because of the volume of beverages you are drinking before you go to bed. I tell patients to stop drinking fluids 2 hours before they go to bed. I don't want people to restrict liquids during the day, especially the elderly, who can get dehydrated; but nighttime is a different story. That late-night soda or coffee may not only keep you up late but is also likely to send you to the bathroom; caffeine is known to increase urine flow.

2 Decrease intake of diuretic medications at night. Some of you may be taking diuretics up to twice a day for conditions such as high blood pressure or congestive heart failure. If that's the case, you might have your doctor consider switching the timing of twice-daily diuretic medications by moving the nighttime dose to late afternoon.

3 Exercise—and by that I mean your Kegel exercises!

4 Manage underlying medical conditions. Remember, diabetes, thyroid disease, multiple sclerosis, and other medical conditions can make urinary problems worse.

when pertaining to your bladder. Much of what we take in our mouths impacts how we get rid of it. Try to remember that caffeine drinks, carbonated beverages, citrus fruits, and even artificial sweeteners can irritate the bladder and cause problems with incontinence.

As I mentioned earlier in the chapter, I find that most people are hesitant to talk with their doctors about urination problems, and many mistakenly think the symptoms they experience are a normal part of aging. Less than half of women and less than 20 percent of men who have urinary problems seek medical treatment. That's a tragedy since urinary problems can significantly impact quality of life. Having urinary problems is associated with depression and work-related absences, and, in the elderly, increases the risks of accidental falls. Our elderly loved ones get up at night to relieve their bladders, they're groggy, maybe a little dizzy, it's dark, and they then trip on the rug in the bathroom. I see the consequences—hip and wrist fractures—all the time. Symptoms of incontinence may also indicate a serious underlying condition such as multiple sclerosis, cancer, or diabetes and should never be dismissed as an age-related inconvenience.

TESTS AND PROCEDURES

If you think you or an elderly relative has urinary problems, what's next? Make an appointment to see your doctor. He or she may perform any of the following tests:

- Basic blood tests to check sugar level, calcium, and kidney function
- Analysis of your urine to check for possible infection, kidney stones, or blood
- Ultrasound to check the urinary system, including the kidneys, the bladder, etc.

Case Study

Amanda is a 60-year-old woman who came in for an appointment with her daughter, Sylvia. Sylvia was concerned because her mother seemed to be "going to the bathroom" far more than usual. Sylvia stated that she had never taken notice of her mother's bathroom usage until the last few months when they were driving to a relative's home and Mom seemed to need to stop every hour and find a restroom.

Amanda seemed to be in overall fair health, but she had not been in for a wellness checkup in nearly 2 years. She has always struggled with her weight—"Sweets are my vice," she says—and she put on more than 40 pounds in the last 5 years. Amanda does admit that for the last year she has been urinating more often than usual. She notes that it also seems to be a larger volume, and she always seems to be thirsty. She gets up at least twice a night to use the bathroom, even after she stopped keeping a glass of water at her bedside.

After completing a physical exam, I ordered some basic blood and urine tests. (She had been fasting.) In the meantime, I asked

Depending on the results of those tests and your particular symptoms, your physician might even perform a stress test for your bladder. During this test, you cough vigorously as the doctor watches for loss of urine from the urinary opening. It may not be the most elegant test, but it can provide useful information.

Help Me Stop Urinating

I'll be honest with you: Urinary problems can be difficult to treat. It's not a condition that's often solved overnight. Sometimes it takes a combination of both behavior changes and medication to achieve success.

So how do we treat urination problems? Again, treatment depends on the particular type of problem, but there are some basic options.

her to document her fluid intake and bathroom visits in a daily log. Her log would later reveal that she was taking in more fluids than normal and was using the bathroom 10 times a day.

The next morning, I received an alert from the lab. Amanda's fasting blood sugar was 210 and her A1c (a measure of how well your blood sugar has been controlled over the last 90 days) was 8 percent. A normal random blood sugar is less than 126, and A1c should be less than 7 percent. Amanda had type 2 diabetes.

I sent Amanda to a diabetes educator, who worked with her on making lifestyle modifications that would help her manage her diabetes. I also prescribed metformin, a drug used to treat diabetes.

Within 2 months, Amanda's blood sugars were almost normal, and her increased urination and increased thirst (two signs of diabetes) had disappeared, now that she had her diabetes under better control. She and Sylvia can now take road trips without using every rest stop they pass by.

Biofeedback. This involves creating a greater awareness of your body and its functions. Biofeedback often uses machines at the beginning to help you identify, locate, and control the pelvic and abdominal muscles. Biofeedback sessions are typically 20 to 30 minutes long, and you may require as many as 10 sessions before you can get the full benefit of this treatment. It takes some practice to get in tune with your body. There truly is a mind-body connection. If you don't believe that now, you will after mastering biofeedback.

Kegels. Most women know about Kegel exercises, which are often touted as one way to make sex more enjoyable. Men typically have not heard about Kegel exercises, think they only apply to women, or simply don't like the whole concept! This is a mistake because when performed correctly, Kegel exercises are often helpful in solving urinary problems because they strengthen the muscles of your pelvic floor, allowing for more control over urinary function.

And best of all, you don't need any equipment or special facility. For men, it's simply a matter of "squeeze, hold, release": When you start urinating, try to stop the flow completely for a few seconds, then release. I tell women to first lie on their backs, and then squeeze the muscles around the vagina and anus. Imagine that muscle like a fist; just as you clench your fist, clench those muscles. Each time you clench, you've performed a Kegel. Once you get used to the exercise, you can do it several times a day.

Medications. There are different types of medications to help with bladder problems, and your doctor will be able to determine the right choice for you. Some of the most common drugs for urinary troubles are anticholinergics. These medications relax bladder muscles and can even help prevent bladder spasms. Remember that medications can also cause urinary problems, so it's important to disclose all medications you're taking to your doctor. Patients often ask me about supplements or natural remedies. In recent years, there's been talk about magnesium, vitamin E, vitamin C, saw palmetto, and pumpkin seeds helping with symptoms. I have to tell you, though, that there are not a lot of studies that support their efficacy, and most patients I treat have not found them to be helpful.

Surgery. There are some surgical options for stress incontinence and overactive bladder. Like any surgery, there are risks and benefits, so you want to be sure to talk with your surgeon about the different types of surgery and how exactly your symptoms might resolve. Surgery is typically recommended only as a last option after other treatments have been found to be ineffective.

Cranberry Juice Doesn't Cure Everything

Remember the movie *My Big Fat Greek Wedding*, where Gus, the father of the bride, uses Windex for all of his ailments? He would spray Windex on wounds and rashes and even housewares, and it seemed to cure any problem. Well, some people seem to think cranberry juice has the same magical healing powers.

The most common belief is that cranberry juice can help treat *urinary tract infections (UTIs)*. UTIs are caused mostly by bacteria. Women get UTIs more often since they have shorter urinary tracts, so bacteria can reach the bladder quicker and easier. Typically, these infections are treated with antibiotics. It's also important to drink plenty of water when you have a UTI.

The truth is there is some good data that shows cranberry juice acidifies the urine and makes it harder for bacteria to stick to the walls of the bladder. Once the bacteria are already on the bladder, the juice doesn't work well in removing them. As a result, it probably is not as helpful for treating an infection as it is for preventing it. So if you like cranberry juice, you should drink it occasionally, and it just might help prevent urinary tract infections. Frequent urinary tract infections are not a normal part of aging. If you suspect that you have a UTI and the symptoms become severe—including fever, back pain, or pain in the side, groin, or belly, as well as blood or pus in the urine—see a doctor immediately, as you may have a kidney infection.

Chapter 5

MEMORIES ARE MADE OF . . . WHAT?

True or False

Memory loss is normal and to be expected
as we get older.   ____

The brain keeps producing new brain cells
until we die.   ____

Normal aging is linked to a loss of intelligence.   ____

You need a CT scan if you have unexplained
memory loss.   ____

(Answers at end of chapter)

Many older—and not so old—adults share a common fear: loss of memory. I'm sure you've been asking yourself some of the typical questions: Is it all right to misplace my keys now and then? Does aging really make it harder to learn and easier to forget, or am I just suffering from information overload? When should I laugh off forgetfulness—and when should I be worried for myself or a loved one? Do those brain-training exercise programs really work?

To answer these questions as well as some others, it is helpful to understand how our brains change as we approach middle age and beyond.

CHANGES IN THE BRAIN AS WE GET OLDER

The brain certainly changes as we age. The brain is an organ, so just like every other organ in your body, it's going to change as you get older. So what are the normal changes?

Well, first of all, the brain does shrink in size; more specifically, the weight of the brain and its volume decrease. Starting around age 25, we gradually lose weight and volume in our brains. The decline is estimated to be about 2 percent per decade. So by the time we are 75, we have lost about 10 percent of our brain size.

That may seem like a lot, but 10 percent is actually not that much of a loss. Not all portions of the brain shrink, or shrink to the same degree; some shrink more than others. For instance, since we are talking about memory, the two areas of the brain that are responsible for memory—the frontal lobe and the hippocampus— typically shrink more than others. That's part of the reason why we develop memory problems.

It is also true that we lose brain cells, called neurons, as we age. How many? Up to 50,000 a day. Don't worry, though, because we have billions of neurons. And that neuron loss occurs throughout our adult lives, not just as we get older.

Some neurons also shrink in size. This matters because their smaller size makes them less effective. They transmit electrical and chemical signals more slowly than they did when we were younger. In addition, as we get older, our bodies make less of the chemicals that our brain cells need to work. That can cause a general slowing of our mental functions.

The grooves on the surface of the brain also widen, while some surface elements become smaller. Just as the blood vessels in the heart develop plaque, the brain also develops plaques and tangles, which in the brain are pieces of dead neurons. These plaques can take up space in living tissue that is responsible for important mental functions, and interfere with your brain's ability to perform these functions.

SOPHISTICATED COMPUTER

Did you have your computer installed by an expert, connecting Internet, video, television, and telephone wires? Have you ever looked behind the computer console? There are so many wires and connections—I have no idea how they all go together. When trying to understand how the brain works, I like to compare it to a sophisticated computer.

The brain is an intricate system of connections. Neurons communicate with one another via chemicals called neurotransmitters. As we age, some connections get lost, and other connections become weaker. This does result in some problems with our thought processes.

The good news is that we can develop new connections even as we get older. The brain is amazingly adaptive and can renew and repair itself. This ability occurs throughout life. Just because brain cells die does not mean that you will automatically experience a significant decline in your mental function. Rather, throughout life, including older age, our brains have both gains and losses, typically keeping everything fairly balanced.

ARE WE GETTING DUMBER?

As we get older, we do not lose intelligence. That is one of the biggest myths—that as we get older, we lose our "smarts." Our cognitive ability typically stays the same in adulthood up through our early sixties. At that point, there is a small decline, but the effects of cognitive changes typically are not noticeable until we reach our seventies and beyond.

Many people continue to gain expertise and skills throughout life. I've known many retirees who got bitten by the travel bug and learned a new language to give them a richer experience. It may take more time to master something like a new language, but older adults still have the ability to do so. Just like computers have a processing speed, so do our brains. With age, our information processing time slows down. This reduced processing time may make it more challenging to multitask. When we're younger, we're able to talk on the phone, type on the computer, and clean our desk—all at the same time! As we get older, we cannot process all of these tasks as quickly or simultaneously.

It is important to point out, though, that new learning can occur at any age—yes, you can teach an old dog new tricks! As a lover of words, I'm happy to tell you that our vocabularies continue to increase throughout our lives, especially if you continue to challenge yourself to read and learn new words.

IS IT NORMAL TO FORGET?

We basically have two types of memory: short-term and long-term. Short-term refers to recent events, such as what you had for dinner last night, what the doctor told you at your recent appointment, or what you read in the newspaper last week. Long-term memory refers to events in the distant past, which is typically defined as remembering details and events that occurred years ago.

Forgetfulness does tend to increase with age. Let me phrase it another way: Memory lapses are a normal part of aging. Everyone forgets things, and occasional short-term memory loss is normal as we get older. That's why you occasionally forget where you put your keys, whether you locked the door, or perhaps what's on television on a Thursday night. It is also normal to occasionally forget an appointment or to forget the names of acquaintances. We all have those "tip of the tongue" moments. Such memory loss is not usually a warning of serious impairment. If you are concerned and aware that you are forgetful at times, that can be a good thing, since folks with dementia often are not aware that they are forgetting.

REVERSIBLE CAUSES OF MEMORY LOSS

If you've ever watched a soap opera, it seems like some character is always suffering from "temporary amnesia" and miraculously regains his or her memory. The truth is, that doesn't happen much in real life, but some causes of memory loss are reversible.

The most common cause of memory loss is medications. Numerous drugs have side effects or interactions with other drugs that can affect memory. Examples include some blood pressure medications, sedatives, and narcotics.

Minor head trauma or injury, such as a concussion, can cause temporary memory loss. Think of the sacked quarterback who is dazed and can't remember for a few moments who he is or where he is. We now know that head injuries, especially on the athletic field, can be quite serious, and the brain needs time to heal. Fortunately, if the injury is minor, the brain does heal and memory returns.

Mental health disorders, especially depression, anxiety, and post-traumatic stress disorder, can cause temporary memory loss and confusion. But if you treat the underlying mental health issue, memory usually returns.

Substance abuse—alcohol and drug use—often can cause memory problems. With alcohol abuse, it's often due to the associated thiamin and B_{12} deficiency. These nutrients are involved in keeping the brain functioning normally, both forming and recalling memories. Marijuana, cocaine, and other drugs block our brain chemicals from creating memories.

Environmental toxins can also cause memory problems; these typically include lead in drinking water or paint, carbon monoxide in home heaters, and chemicals in various pesticides and home cleaning materials. Have you ever tried to breathe in the bathroom after a thorough cleaning with various chemicals? It definitely can make you woozy!

Infection is a major cause of older persons becoming confused and disoriented. Again, this usually happens suddenly. Once the infection is treated, the person returns to normal.

Some overlooked causes of memory loss include dehydration, which can be quite common in the elderly, as well as thyroid problems. Sometimes people are either over- or undermedicated on thyroid replacement, and this causes some memory problems and confusion. Poorly controlled diabetes can also cause problems with your thoughts and memory. (Try appearing normal when your blood sugar is dangerously low or high—I bet you can't!) Hearing loss is another overlooked area that is mistaken for brain problems. Too often, people cannot hear what was said, they are too embarrassed to ask someone to repeat it, and then they cannot remember it because they never heard it in the first place!

Finally, the hospital setting itself can actually cause confusion and memory loss, especially as we get older. It is a strange setting that disrupts sleep patterns, and new medications are typically started, often narcotics. As anyone who has ever had a baby knows, lack of sleep can cause mental confusion and temporary memory loss and forgetfulness—and hospitals can be tough places to get a good night's sleep.

WHEN SHOULD I BE CONCERNED?

There is a big difference between normal absentmindedness and the types of memory loss associated with dementia such as

Alzheimer's. Some forgetfulness and slowing of mental responses are a normal part of aging. After all, aging affects memory by changing the way the brain stores information and thereby makes it harder to recall stored memories. However, significant memory loss is not a normal part of aging.

So what's considered "significant" memory loss? When evaluating the seriousness of memory loss, you want to determine whether the forgetfulness is gradual (over many months to years) or sudden (several days, weeks, or a couple of months). If memory loss is sudden, it's typically not related to Alzheimer's. Normal memory loss is not sudden, and it doesn't significantly worsen over time; dementia also starts slowly but gets much worse over several months to several years. Sudden memory loss is usually related to one of the reversible causes mentioned earlier.

Some "red flags" that should raise concern for you or a loved one include:

- Trouble remembering how to do things you've done many times before, such as driving to your favorite restaurant, playing golf, or loading songs onto your iPod
- Forgetting things much more often than you used to, such that you are forgetting something every day

Memory: What's Normal and Not Normal As We Age

Normal	Not Normal
Occasional memory loss of recent events	Loss of long-term memories
Difficulty multitasking efficiently	Gradual, progressive memory loss
Needing more time to get a job or task done	Unable to complete simple tasks or name family members
"Tip of the tongue" moments	Sudden memory loss

- Trouble learning new things such as a new computer skill
- Difficulty following directions effectively
- Trouble handling money
- Repeating phrases or stories in the same conversation
- Appearing disheveled/unkempt, with changes in grooming

Exhibiting any of these symptoms should prompt medical attention.

ALZHEIMER'S DISEASE

Alzheimer's is a disease of the brain that affects our memory as well as our thinking and behavior. It is the most common form of dementia. Unfortunately, it is not reversible and gets progressively worse over time.

Alzheimer's is not a normal part of aging. In fact, no type of dementia should be considered normal. Contrary to what you may have been told, we do not become senile just because we get older.

Symptoms of Alzheimer's typically first include memory loss, and then progress to changes in thinking and then finally behavior. Typically, early Alzheimer's disease causes a person to be unable to complete tasks that are familiar. An example would be when the person gets lost while driving on familiar streets and routes. Misplacing your car keys is normal, but if you misplace keys in an inappropriate place—such as the freezer—that should raise an alarm. Because Alzheimer's affects short-term memory at first, those developing the disease often ask the same questions over and over, since they cannot retain the answer. They are less able to follow directions; you often see this when they cannot follow a recipe, even if in the past they were an excellent cook.

As Alzheimer's progresses, patients start to mix up words because their memory problems impact their thinking ability. They use the wrong word or have difficulty remembering common words (e.g., a pen or a clock). They often undergo personality changes, resulting in unusual behaviors. As the disease worsens, they become unable to take care of themselves, unable to perform what we call activities of daily living (e.g., eating, bathing, walking, climbing stairs, grooming). Finally, long-term memory is impacted, but that's usually the last cognition to be affected.

Although most people are quite fearful of Alzheimer's, only 6 percent of those in their sixties are affected by the disease. It rarely affects anyone in their forties or fifties, and it is highly unlikely you or a loved one has Alzheimer's if you're not at least 60. The incidence does increase each decade after 60, and with our aging population, more people will develop Alzheimer's. Approximately 30 percent of people will have some degree of Alzheimer's by the time they are over 85.

EXAM TIME

If you are concerned about memory loss—whether for yourself or a loved one—you should see your doctor, and possibly a neurologist. You will undergo neuropsychological testing and will likely need a CT scan, PET scan, or MRI.

One of the simplest tests that you can administer to a loved one, or have someone administer to you, is the mini-mental status exam. Physicians will give you this test if they suspect dementia, but there's no reason why you can't also administer this test to someone else (if you're concerned about your own memory loss, ask someone to administer it to you).

The MMSE,[1] also referred to as the Folstein test, is a brief 30-point questionnaire that doctors often use to screen for dementia. It can also help a doctor determine the severity of any cognitive impairment. The questionnaire takes about 10 to 15 minutes to complete and basically focuses on the following areas: orientation, registration, attention and calculation, recall, and language.

Orientation

What is the year? Season? Date? Day? Month? _____

One point for each correct answer. Maximum score of 5.

Where are we?
State? County? Town? Hospital/Building? Floor/Room? _____

One point for each correct answer. Maximum score of 5.

Registration

Name three unrelated objects (e.g., fast car, blue ball, button), taking 1 second for each. Then ask the patient to repeat all three objects after you have said them.

This first attempt determines the patient's score (out of 3), but keep saying them until the patient can repeat all three.

_____

Attention and Calculation

Ask the patient to begin with 100 and count backward by 7. We call these "serial sevens." Stop after five subtractions (93, 86, 79, 72 ,65).

Score the total number of correct answers. _____
An alternative is to spell the word "world" backward.

The score is the number of letters in correct order, e.g., dlrow = 5; dlorw = 2.

Recall

Ask the patient if he/she can recall the three words you previously asked him/her to remember.

Score 1 for each correct answer. _____

Language

Naming: Show the patient a wristwatch and ask him or her what it is. Repeat for pencil.

Score 1 for each correct answer. _____

Repetition: Ask the patient to repeat a sentence after you. Allow only one trial.

Score 1 if the repetition is completely correct and zero if it is not. _____

3-Stage Command: State a command first and then give the patient a piece of plain blank paper.

Score 1 point for each part correctly executed. _____

Reading: On a blank piece of paper print the sentence "Close your eyes" in letters large enough for the patient to see clearly. Ask him or her to read it and do what it says.

Score 1 point only if he actually closes his or her eyes. _____

Writing: Give the patient a blank piece of paper and ask him or her to write a sentence for you.

Do not dictate a sentence; it is to be written spontaneously. It must contain a subject and verb and be sensible. _____

Copying: On a clean piece of paper, draw intersecting pentagons, with each side about 1 inch, and ask him or her to copy it exactly as it is.

All 10 angles must be present and two must intersect to score 1 point. _____

Scoring

25–30 Normal   **10–20 Moderate Dementia**
21–24 Mild Dementia   **< 9 Severe Dementia**

Remember, this is a screening tool. If the results are not normal, more testing might be required.

PREVENTION

I wish I had some more information to share with you here. There is some good evidence that a healthy diet as well as exercise—both physical and mental—can help reduce or delay memory loss and possibly Alzheimer's.

Physical exercise can be as simple as walking. A recent study shows that walking about a mile a day—or 6 miles a week—appears to maintain brain volume and preserve memory in old age.

FOUR TIPS TO HELP YOU REMEMBER

1 Write things down. Keep lists and make journal entries. Maintain a detailed calendar. Use self-adhesive notes and put them on a door or mirror. If you need to remember something important, it doesn't hurt to write it down, and then put that piece of paper where you'll see it. Just consider it to be a gentle reminder.

2 Establish routines and follow them. I always put my office keys in my briefcase right after I open the door. I don't put them on the desk or in my pocket. That way, I always know where they are.

3 Make associations and connections. This means a couple of things. If you can link an event or a memory to another event or memory, you'll be more likely to remember it, since you've established connections in your brain. For example, you might associate the first name of a colleague at your company to the name of a best friend from high school. Or you might connect the route to your favorite restaurant with the route to your child's school. The more connections you make to events or facts, the more you'll increase the chances that you'll remember them later in life.

Similarly, I also recommend being socially connected. Remember, depression can cause memory problems; if you become more socially connected, you are less likely to become depressed.

4 Stay active both physically and mentally.

Case Study

As I look back on it, I think the first time I briefly thought about Alzheimer's in my father was probably when he got lost while driving me to the airport one day. He must have driven that route at least a hundred times, so I was a bit surprised when he started to get confused about which road to turn onto. I attributed it to him being distracted. But the second time it happened, a few months later, caused me to pause. After all, my father was not only an excellent driver but he was always precise; he was a "numbers guy"—an accountant by training who always seemed to be doing calculations. So a driving error was quite imprecise. It didn't happen every time he drove me, but it happened enough times that I started to get a little concerned. About a year after those incidents, he started to get lost in the neighborhood. At that time, we just attributed it to him getting older, not thinking it was that serious.

As the months progressed, I noticed other changes, mostly small at first. I will admit it: My father seemed to be getting a bit moody as he got older. But we all figured that some mood changes were to be expected with retirement. Like a lot of men of his generation, my father worked hard to support his family. He even worked two jobs for a time to help pay tuition costs for college and medical school. So my father never really developed too many hobbies (golf wasn't the "in" thing to do back then, but he did like to bowl sometimes!), and we all attributed some moodiness to boredom. He did, however, light up when spending time with his grandchildren.

Reading books, newspapers, and magazines, doing crossword puzzles and games like Sudoku, watching educational television shows, and participating in hobbies may all help keep your brain as sharp as possible. These strategies have not been proven to prevent or delay the onset of dementia, but they are likely to help keep older minds sharp.

I started to get more concerned when my father started to repeat certain words and phrases that did not make sense. This was highly unusual since my father was a very smart man. He rarely made grammatical errors. Nonetheless, it's hard for a family to think about the diagnosis of Alzheimer's, knowing all the emotions that go along with such a diagnosis.

My mother eventually took him to a neurologist, who did neuropsychological testing, and indeed he was given a diagnosis of Alzheimer's. At first, my father was very upset by his forgetfulness, but as the disease progressed, it didn't seem to bother him. He seemed to be unaware of it. Over the next couple of years, my father—always accompanied by my mother and often my sister—was in and out of the doctor's office, trying different medications to treat memory loss (none of which seemed to help) as well as symptoms of agitation and sleeplessness (some success). Ultimately, his condition rapidly deteriorated over 3 years, which is a bit unusual for Alzheimer's. Often, it's a long process, known as the long good-bye. Our family decided to keep him at home and arranged home hospice. In the end, my father was able to die peacefully at home, surrounded by his family.

I'm not sure if recognizing his symptoms earlier and being given the label of Alzheimer's would have made much difference in my father's care, given where we are, or more accurately where we are not, with treatment options. I do believe, however, that early diagnosis can encourage some families to spend more time with loved ones now before it gets too late.

You probably have seen various supplements and vitamins being promoted to improve memory and prevent Alzheimer's. We just don't have any good information to suggest that they do; some supplements and vitamins have other beneficial health effects, but don't take or buy one simply to improve memory.

Finally, manage any medical conditions such as high blood

pressure, heart disease, and diabetes, which can increase your risk of stroke and cause memory loss and brain problems.

GENETIC TEST FOR ALZHEIMER'S DISEASE

There are currently some genetic tests that can tell you if you're at risk genetically to develop Alzheimer's. But it's important to remember that genetics is just one component of your risk of developing Alzheimer's. Even if you are at risk, it does not mean you will develop it. In addition, we currently do not have any truly effective therapies to delay or cure Alzheimer's. So when patients ask me if they should have a genetic test, I ask them, "What would you do with the information?" That answer is intensely personal: Every person has to decide for him or herself how to live and plan for the rest of their life.

ROLE OF CAREGIVERS

I would be remiss if I did not mention the role of caregivers in a chapter that discusses Alzheimer's. Many of you reading this book are or have been a caregiver for an elderly parent at some point. Nearly one out of every four households provides care to a relative age 50 or older. What is particularly impressive is that the average age of a primary caregiver is 60 years old—and as you'd suspect, nearly 75 percent of them are women. (I always tell couples planning to have a baby that one of the major factors in *not* being admitted to a nursing home is having a daughter.)

I really consider these caregivers to be heroes. It is an enormously challenging job. Caregivers often experience a sense of burden, and some researchers estimate that nearly 50 percent are depressed. Many are sleep deprived and exhausted. I've seen the physical and emotional toll it can take on numerous family members and friends. Given their age, the lack of sleep often exacerbates their own health problems. They really are the "hidden patient," and we need to do a better job of focusing on their care as well.

Answers to true/false statements: True, True, False, True

Chapter 6

SEEING CLEARLY

True or False

Floaters in the eye are common once we reach age 50. _____

Pupils become smaller as we age. _____

If you live long enough, you will develop a cataract. _____

Chances are you'll need reading glasses by the time you're 55. _____

(Answers at end of chapter)

Have you ever heard "The eyes are the window to the soul"? I don't know about seeing the soul, but the eyes do tell us a great deal about our overall health. If you understand what happens to your vision as you age, you'll learn a lot about changes in your other body functions as well.

I find that people often say vision is one of the most important senses. Some people's greatest fear is losing their ability to see. When my sister wanted me to believe something she said while we were growing up, she'd often say, "I swear on my eyes." I still didn't believe her half the time, but it did make a statement about how important vision is to her.

Think of our eyes working just like a camera. I don't mean the sort of point-and-shoot camera that has become so commonplace

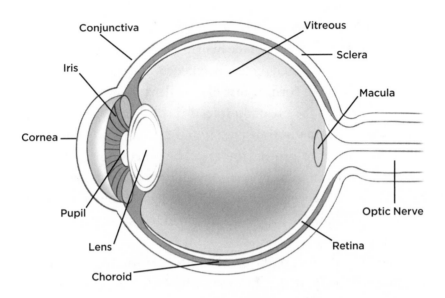

Anatomy of the Eye—The eye is actually a fluid-filled ball, with the cornea and lens *(left)* at the front of your eye and the optic nerve *(right)* connecting the back of the eye to the brain.

in today's world, but rather the type of camera we used growing up. Surely, you remember awkwardly adjusting a lens and positioning people in the frame. And your photos probably still came out a little out-of-focus and off-center.

A visual aid—no pun intended—is probably useful at this point. See above for an illustration of the anatomy of the eye.

SOPHISTICATED CAMERAS

Like a good camera, the eye has several components that affect your view, including the sclera, cornea, pupil, iris, lens, retina, optic nerve, and conjunctiva. If anything goes wrong with one of these components, we have trouble seeing.

"Don't fire until you see the whites of their eyes" was a command supposedly made famous at the Battle of Bunker Hill during the American Revolution. I suppose it does sound much more dramatic than "Don't fire until you see their sclera," but either way, it's the same thing. The white part of the human eye is called the sclera, and it serves as the eye's tough protective outer covering.

Next comes the cornea. Just like the lens cover on a camera, the cornea covers the eye and protects the delicate parts beneath. The cornea is actually transparent and contains two layers. Its outer layer helps to protect the eye. The inner layer is the part where light first hits the eye. As a result, the cornea is primarily responsible for focusing—it bends rays of light through the pupil. I'm sure you know the pupil—it's the small black circle in the middle of the eye.

The iris is the part of the eye that often gets the most attention, because it is the part that has the distinctive color that so often serves as an identification trademark for people. It's the iris that allows us to say a romantic interest has big, beautiful brown eyes! But the iris serves a much more important purpose than simply looking pretty. It also acts like the aperture of a camera, controlling how much light passes into the eye by dilating and constricting the pupil.

To see how the iris and the pupil work together, go into a dark room and remain in the dark for several seconds, then turn the lights on suddenly. When the lights are off, your pupils will dilate (get bigger) to allow more light to come in, but when the lights come on suddenly, they are literally overwhelmed with light, which sometimes can cause some visual discomfort. You will find yourself having trouble adjusting to the sudden brightness, because it will take a moment or two for your iris to get the message to your pupils to contract (get smaller). Remember the trapped miners in Chile? When they were rescued after 70 days underground, they were all wearing sunglasses when they came back to the surface, to protect their eyes from the bright lights at the scene until their irises and pupils could readjust. It was not meant to be a fashion statement.

The lens of the eye, as you'd expect, acts like the lens in the camera, helping to focus light to the back of the eye. It actually changes shape to achieve clear focus.

At the back of the eye is a layer known as the retina. The macula is a small region in the center of the retina, and it's responsible for central vision as well as the ability to distinguish some colors. Think of the macula as the viewfinder and the retina as the film of the camera. The retina's purpose is basically to record what it is you are looking at in the form of vision. How does it do this? Well, the retina has numerous photoreceptor nerve cells that change the light rays into electrical impulses. These impulses are then sent through the optic nerve (which has more than a million nerve fibers) to the brain, which welcomes the images like a proud grandparent receiving pictures of a grandchild. The whole process occurs in milliseconds.

Like a sophisticated camera, the eye is impacted by wear and tear. Our vision is actually one of the first functions affected as we get older. You may have already noticed a decrease in vision starting in your late teens. Major changes start to occur again typically after age 40.

SMALLER PUPILS

As we get older, our pupils become smaller and our field of vision decreases. The lens also becomes more rigid. As a result, our ability to focus on objects both near and far becomes more difficult. In addition, our vision becomes less sharp. You probably have noticed this because it's hard to read fine print. This usually starts to occur in our forties. If you get headaches or your eyes seem to get tired after reading small print, you may have presbyopia. *Presbyopia* is the medical term for the loss of elasticity of the lens, which results in loss of sharp focus for near objects, and it is a normal part of aging. You probably remember your parents or grandparents wearing reading glasses or bifocals—presbyopia is why they needed them, and now you may need them too.

You probably have also noticed that you need more light to read clearly as you've gotten older. I've noticed this when I'm in a nice restaurant. The restaurant is usually dimly lit, which can provide a nice atmosphere but makes it tough to read the menu or decipher the numbers on the bill when it arrives. This challenge is normal because as you get older, you need more light to see. So go ahead and move those candles closer to the bill so you can read it...and make sure your waitress gets a nice tip!

VISION CHANGES IN THE ELDERLY

If you're caring for elderly patients, it's important to remember that it's harder for them to read smaller words and numbers. Be sure to write emergency numbers or special instructions larger than you normally would do. I recommend to my elderly patients that they mention their vision issues to their local pharmacy; the pharmacist can print labels and instructions in larger print. It's also a good idea to get a cell phone for them that has large buttons and numbers.

MORE LIGHT

If you're living with elderly loved ones, you might want to consider installing additional light, especially night-lights in various rooms, such as their bedroom as well as bathrooms. Consider adding more light in stairways, too. I often recommend that night-lights be placed in the hallway since more light is necessary to ensure safety. You want to avoid falls, which can then lead to serious medical problems.

FLOATERS

Many middle-aged patients come to see me about a common problem called floaters. This refers to the experience of seeing spots or specks that float across the visual field. They can be very scary, especially the first time they occur. However, they are usually normal. To understand floaters, it's helpful to learn about the vitreous.

The vitreous is a jellylike substance that fills the body of the eye. It's attached to the retina, and is typically clear. However, as we age, it becomes less jellylike and more waterlike. Sometimes it even detaches from the retina. The floaters are actually little clumps of the jelly-type substance, which then cast shadows. Again, this is usually normal and most floaters resolve on their own over time. However, if the onset of floaters coincides with a flash of light, or seems to be associated with any sudden physical

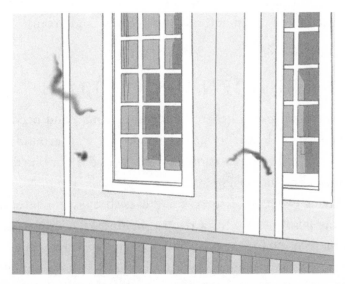

Floaters—These small spots that float through our visual field are especially noticeable when we look at a blank and/or light-colored surface, such as the blue sky. These can be normal if minimally visible, but when more severe, they can be associated with eye strain, retinal tear, and other eye ailments.

weakness, see your doctor, as these symptoms can indicate a retinal detachment or even a stroke.

The illustration on page 99 will help you to understand how a floater obstructs your vision.

COLOR BLINDNESS

Have you been worried that you seem to have lost some of your ability to discern the difference between colors, or different shades of the same color? Maybe when you're at a store and take your black sweater to the register, you suddenly realize that it's actually blue. While we don't become color-blind as we become older, our ability to distinguish greens and blues can be affected. This is because the lens of the eye begins to yellow with age. You may have even noticed this while watching television or looking at photos. It typically does not happen until after age 50, and generally does not cause major problems. Luckily, traffic lights are red, yellow, and green and not blue, yellow, and green!

SUDDEN VISION LOSS

Sudden vision loss is never normal at any age, and needs to be evaluated by a doctor immediately. Do not wait around hoping that it will get better. If vision suddenly goes dark or blurry, get to the emergency room right away.

Having eye pain or severely red eyes that last for several days in a row is also cause for a trip to the doctor, as these could be symptoms of a more serious condition. Just because you get older doesn't mean you should have pain in the eye like you might in a knee or shoulder. Same goes for redness. Neither of these is normal, and they need to be evaluated.

COMMON EYE CONDITIONS

There are many elderly persons who experience only minor vision changes well into their eighties. But it's worthwhile to look at some of the common eye conditions that may occur as we age. All of these should be evaluated since they are not to be considered part of the normal aging process. Too often, when people think symptoms are part of normal aging, they ignore them, and thereby sometimes ignore an underlying disease, which can result in permanent deterioration of vision. There are often successful treatments available and even some ways to prevent or delay certain conditions.

Cataracts

There's a mistaken belief that everyone will develop a cataract if he or she lives long enough. The truth is that less than 20 percent of persons younger than 75 years have a cataract. As we age, the lens can become cloudy, and vision then becomes blurry and hazy. When the lens becomes cloudy, less light passes through, and vision decreases. People with cataracts often describe a feeling as if there's a fog over the eye. Colors may appear faded as well. It is important to keep in mind that pain and redness are not common symptoms of cataracts. Cataracts form slowly, so these symptoms can evolve over a year or two. Be on the lookout for this cloudiness, because cataracts can be treated fairly easily these days with surgery. See your doctor if your vision is becoming cloudy.

Detached Retina

The retina is the thin membrane of nerves that lines the back of the eye (see page 95 for diagram). As the name of the condition implies, the retina can actually become separated from the rest of the eye

FIVE TIPS TO IMPROVE EYE HEALTH

1 Wear sunglasses. Not only are your eyes more sensitive to light as you get older, they also are more affected by wind and particles in the air. Sunglasses can help serve as a barrier to protect your eyes from the elements.

2 Get a yearly eye exam. You need to make sure that your doctor puts drops in your eyes to dilate your pupils. You may remember having to wear dark glasses after an exam in the past. This is because your pupils get bigger when they are dilated, and bright light will make it difficult to see until your pupils return to normal size. Dilation is important for the eye doctor to get a really good look at your eyes.

3 Supplement. I don't mean just eating carrots, but your mother was right—the beta-carotene in carrots does support eye health. As we get older, it's harder to get all of the necessary nutrients from our diets. Therefore, I suggest to many patients that they consider taking 50 milligrams daily of beta-carotene, 500 milligrams daily of vitamin C, 400 international units of vitamin E, and 80 milligrams of zinc.

4 Limit time in front of screens. We spend too many hours in front of our computers, televisions, video games, and our mobile devices. Staring too long at screens causes eye strain. The longer you have to focus

tissue. You might have heard or read about boxers or other athletes who have experienced a detached retina—usually from being hit in the eye. Most detachments, however, are not caused by trauma or injury, but are the result of an underlying condition that makes you more susceptible to detachment. These include severe nearsightedness, glaucoma, and prior eye surgery, such as cataract surgery. Poorly controlled diabetes can also put you at risk. As you'd suspect, the odds of experiencing retinal detachment increase as you age.

on a screen, the harder your eye muscles have to work to keep it in focus. Try to spend no more than 1 uninterrupted hour in front of a screen.

5 Exercise your eyes. Some researchers believe that when we wear corrective lenses, our eyes become weaker because they do not need to make any effort to focus clearly; in a sense, we develop a dependency on our glasses and contacts when we wear them continuously. I recommend a couple of different eye exercises to keep your eyes challenged.

The first one is to roll your eyes. I'm sure you've done that at some point in your life, usually when you're bored with someone or something. You do it simply by slowly rolling your eyes in a circular, clockwise direction. Then, move them back in a counterclockwise direction. Do this several times a day for about 1 minute. Another good exercise is to focus both eyes on your left index finger. Then, slowly move your finger straight out away from your nose until you reach arm's length. Bring your finger in close, and then slowly move it back out again. Next, move your finger to the left so it's parallel to your shoulder. Keep your eyes focused on it. Don't move your head as you watch your moving finger. Instead, use and exercise your eye muscles. Repeat the steps with your right index finger. Again, do this several times a day for at least 1 minute.

If your retina becomes detached, you'll know it—you'll usually see flashing lights, which some people describe as streaks of lightning along the edges of the visual field. You may also see floaters. Sometimes you will see a persistent shadow across your visual field.

Early diagnosis and repair are critical. You typically will need surgery. Left untreated, a retinal detachment can lead to blindness.

It's hard to prevent retinal detachment. Obviously, you want to

Vision: What's Normal and Not Normal As We Age	
Normal	**Not Normal**
Difficulty reading fine print	Sudden change in vision
Floaters	Redness and pain
Difficulty seeing in the dark	Color blindness
Occasional blurriness near end of day	Blurriness with glasses or contact lenses

avoid injury to the eye, and if you do get injured, you want to be on the lookout for signs of detachment. If you're involved in racquet sports like squash, I do recommend protective eyeglasses.

Glaucoma

Glaucoma is the result of either too much fluid production in the eye or a blockage that causes pressure to build up and do damage to the optic nerve. Common symptoms include blurred vision as well as halos. Sometimes there is also eye pain. Many times, however, there are no early symptoms of glaucoma. Often the pressure builds up slowly, and symptoms are gradual. By the time symptoms become noticeable, glaucoma may be in a late stage.

To prevent glaucoma or to treat it in the early stages, it is critical that you have an annual eye exam after you reach age 40. Your eye doctor should measure the pressure in your eyes to screen for this disease. During this exam, you must hold your eye wide open, and a small device will actually reach into your eye and touch it. This can be a little uncomfortable for some people, but it's an essential screening test and well worth the temporary discomfort.

The good news is that there are several treatments for glaucoma. These include surgery, eye drops, and oral medications. The key is early detection.

Macular Degeneration

As mentioned earlier, the macula is a small area of the retina responsible for fine acute vision. Degeneration of the macula typically presents as loss of central vision. If you have macular degeneration, you might feel like you are experiencing "tunnel vision" or you might feel like your visual field is closing in. Many patients will complain of losing sharp vision such that words on a page or a sign sometimes appear bent or wavy, or that objects appear smaller.

Macular degeneration is the most common cause of blindness for people over the age of 55. Other risk factors include high blood pressure, high cholesterol, smoking, and obesity. Genetics also plays an important role—in fact, if a first-degree relative, such as

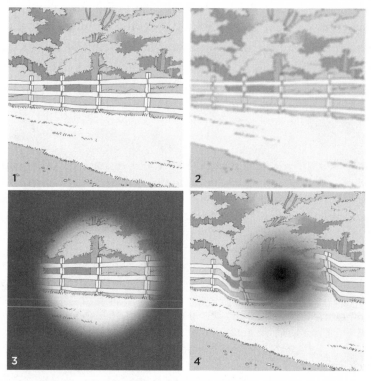

Eye Disease Impact on Vision—(1) Normal vision, (2) Near-sighted means objects far away appear blurry and not in perfect focus, (3) Vision with glaucoma is likened to "looking through a straw," and (4) Macular degeneration causes a distortion of the center of the visual field.

a parent or sibling, has suffered from macular degeneration, you have a 50 percent chance of developing the condition. If you do have a family history of this disease, it's important to vigilantly monitor for early symptoms, and see your doctor immediately if you become concerned.

There are two types of macular degeneration: dry and wet. Dry macular degeneration occurs when light-sensitive cells in the macula break down. This is a slow process that results in blurry central vision, and over time, central vision is lost completely. Wet is the more serious type, but it can be successfully treated if it is diagnosed early. Treatment involves medicine as well as laser surgery. In wet macular degeneration, abnormal blood vessels from the retina actually start to grow under the macula. These blood vessels break easily, leaking blood and other fluids. That causes the macula to bulge from a position that is meant to be flat, causing us to lose our central vision focus. Usually folks also see dark spots in their vision and straight lines look wavy. Without treat-

Case Study

Julie is a 70-year-old patient with heart disease and diabetes who routinely comes to appointments with her younger sister, Lisa. On a recent visit, Lisa remarked that Julie had bumped into a doorway a couple of times over the past few months. They both thought it might be due to a new blood pressure medication Julie had started taking.

I examined Julie's gait, and it seemed fine. I also asked about dizziness, which can result from blood pressure medications. Julie said she didn't have any dizziness. But then she said that sometimes the "doorway seemed crooked." I suspected a potential vision problem. Julie confessed that over the last year, people's faces sometimes seemed a bit wavy, but she thought that was just because "I need a new eyeglass prescription, Dr. Whyte, and I just haven't gotten around to seeing my eye doctor."

Although I don't do extensive eye exams, I knew this was a concern. I immediately referred Julie to an ophthalmologist

ment, both types of macular degeneration lead to permanent vision loss. Since the symptoms appear gradually, make sure to tell your doctor at your annual eye exam about any changes in the clearness of your vision.

Diabetes and the Eye

Given the increasing incidence of diabetes—especially due to obesity—it is important to mention diabetic retinopathy. As its name implies, this disease of the retina is caused by diabetes. In this condition, small blood vessels stop supplying blood to the retina. Sometimes, these blood vessels leak fluid, which can make it difficult to see clearly. As the disease progresses, new blood vessels (which are often abnormal and fragile) grow to supply the retina with blood. New growth may sound good, but it actually is not in this case, since the new vessels send blood to the center of the eye—the wrong place. This condition can usually be treated effectively with laser therapy.

friend she could see the same day. Although it wasn't truly urgent, I knew that Julie doesn't make going to the eye doctor a priority. "She much prefers going to her cardiologist. He's cuter," Lisa once remarked.

After Julie saw the eye doctor, she was diagnosed with acute macular degeneration in the right eye. And she had the more serious "wet type." Luckily, she was able to get photodynamic therapy. After 3 months, her vision was not completely restored, but it was better, and she stopped bumping into doorways.

Julie had several of the risk factors for macular degeneration: She was over 60, she had high blood pressure, and she had high cholesterol. And she had symptoms, but she thought her vision changes were a "normal" part of aging, when they definitely were not. Too often, people don't think about making going to the eye doctor annually a priority. It's important to see a specialist for your eye care, not just your family doctor.

Pinkeye (Conjunctivitis)

It seems as if everyone at some point has had conjunctivitis—more commonly known as pinkeye. The conjunctiva is a thin lining over the sclera, the white part of the eye. In medical terminology, the suffix "itis" usually implies associated inflammation or swelling. So, conjunctivitis is inflammation of the conjunctiva. Cells in the conjunctiva produce mucus, which helps to lubricate the eye. When an infection or allergy is present, the conjunctiva becomes inflamed and turns red or pink, and your eye produces more of the lubricating mucus to soothe itself. Patients sometimes say they feel like they have sand in their eyes. Pinkeye is much more common in children than adults, but it can occur in the elderly. It is fairly harmless, but if it is due to infection, it is very contagious and should be treated immediately with antibiotics.

Dry Eye

People often notice changes in tearing as they age. Dry eye is a condition that usually results from a blocked tear duct, which decreases our ability to make tears and can lead to itching and burning. Dry eye can also cause you to tear excessively, since your eyes may overproduce tears to make up for the blocked duct. None of these symptoms are normal—they can be a sign of infection and should be evaluated by a doctor. Your doctor can actually do a test to measure the amount of tears you produce. And no, women do not produce more tears than men—except maybe at the movies!

Answers to true/false statements: True, True, False, True

Chapter 7

CAN YOU HEAR ME NOW?

True or False

Most people need a hearing aid by age 70. _____

We all experience some hearing loss as we age. _____

Listening to loud music as a teenager will result in hearing loss later in life. _____

You might need an MRI if you have sudden hearing loss. _____

If you have hearing loss in only one ear, it's usually not serious. _____

(Answers at end of chapter)

I know you've seen those commercials for a wireless phone company with the gentleman walking all around the country saying, "Can you hear me now?" Well, depending upon how old you are, you might have some trouble hearing him no matter what cell phone carrier you're using! The reality is that we all experience some hearing loss as we age. It's a normal part of getting older.

Hearing loss is a common problem that we all experience occasionally. I'm certain you attended a rock concert when you

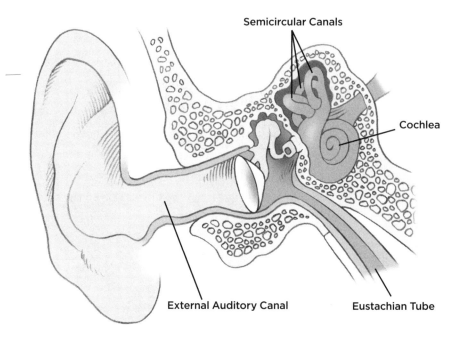

Semicircular Canals

Cochlea

External Auditory Canal

Eustachian Tube

Anatomy of the Ear—Cross section through the side of the head, showing the ear and ear canal leading into the skull where the inner ear lies. The ear drum is connected to the small bones to its right called the ossicles, which transmit vibrations farther inward where they are transformed into electrical impulses the brain can comprehend.

were younger and had trouble hearing the next day. You also might have experienced hearing loss as the result of an infection. All of these are temporary and can occur at any age.

To understand how hearing changes as we age, let's review how the ear works. The ears may be small, but they're quite powerful.

Think of the ear as having three segments:

1. **Outer ear.** This consists of the auricle and ear.
2. **Inner ear.** This includes the semicircular canals, cochlea, and internal auditory canals.
3. **Middle ear.** This comprises the tympanic membrane, ossicles, and the middle ear space.

It's important to understand how your ears work, so that you can determine whether your hearing loss is a normal part of aging or a sign of a more serious condition.

HOW WE HEAR SOUND

Would you believe hair actually allows us to hear? That's right—tiny hairs inside your ears help you hear. The outer ear catches sound waves (which are actually vibrations of the air) and funnels them down the external auditory canal. The hairs pick up the sound waves and change them into nerve signals that the brain interprets as sound. Each hair cell is serviced by more than 20 neurons. Different groups of hair cells are responsible for high versus low frequencies. Hearing loss occurs when the tiny hairs inside the ear are damaged or die. The problem is that unlike the hair on our heads, hair cells in our ears do not regrow, so when hairs are damaged or die, the resulting hearing loss is usually permanent.

Some hearing loss is normal and a natural part of aging; we even have a word for it—*presbycusis*. As we age, several things happen: The cochlea becomes less flexible and more rigid; the auditory nerve becomes worn out; and numerous hair cells have died. All of this contributes to hearing loss. At first, it becomes difficult to hear high-frequency sounds, such as someone talking. The son or daughter of an elderly patient will often comment that the television volume is quite loud in their home. Or a wife will tell me she has to shout at her husband or repeat what she has said to get a response. (I know, I know . . . hearing loss isn't the only reason some husbands don't respond.) As hearing gets worse, it may become more difficult to hear sounds at lower pitches as well, such as the radio or someone speaking in a deep voice.

Most hearing loss does not become noticeable, however, until we're in our sixties. And it typically gets worse each decade after age 60. By the time we approach age 70, nearly half of us will have some hearing loss. And age-related hearing loss typically occurs in both ears, not just one. As you would expect, normal hearing loss occurs gradually over the years. Rapid or sudden hearing loss is never normal.

DOES BLASTING MUSIC REALLY HURT?

Heredity plays an important role in determining whether you will develop significant hearing loss. So if your parents and grandparents had hearing problems, you will be more likely to lose some hearing as well.

But there are other risk factors for hearing loss aside from heredity and age. If you once held a job in which you were exposed to a lot of noise on a daily basis, you're more likely to experience hearing problems as you get older. I'm not talking about kindergarten teachers who are around screaming kids all day, but construction workers and airplane mechanics who are exposed to constant loud levels of noise. And it is true that if you blast the music in your ears through your iPod or other headphones, you are likely causing damage that will manifest itself years later. Repeat ear infections can also cause hearing problems later in life. We're not yet sure why, but diabetes, high blood pressure, osteoporosis, and even smoking can also cause hearing problems or make them worse, so it's important to watch your overall health to maximize your hearing.

HOW LOUD IS TOO LOUD?

What we think of as "loudness" is often subjective. My wife always turns down the radio in the car, for instance, while I keep turning it up. (That may also be because we like different music!) But there are some general guidelines that can help you determine when a sound might be too loud and therefore dangerous to your hearing. When evaluating sounds, I always tell patients to think of sound in three ways: (1) How loud is it? (2) How long are you exposed to it? and (3) How close are you to it?

Sound is measured in a unit called decibels. As a rule, scientists warn that exposure to sound higher than 110 decibels for more than 60 seconds can risk permanent hearing loss. They also recommend that you should not be exposed to more than 15 minutes of unprotected exposure of 100 decibels. And prolonged exposure—more than 2 hours—to any noise above 90 decibels can cause gradual hearing loss.

I know, you're thinking who's going to carry around a sound level meter to know how loud something is? (I actually did walk around with a sound level meter for several weeks in sixth grade as part of a science fair project; I received a lot of strange looks.) The chart below will help you get a sense of the loudness of the sounds you're regularly exposed to.

Activity	Decibel Level
Whisper	20
Normal conversation	60
Washing machine	75
Dial tone	80
Lawn mower, hair dryer	90
Headphones at volume level 5 of 10	100
Chain saw	110
Leaf blower	115
Ambulance	120
Rock concert, fireworks	140
Shotgun, jet engine	155

Did you notice that listening to music at a level of 5 (out of 10) through your headphones generates sound at 100 decibels? That can cause permanent hearing loss if you listen at that level more than 15 minutes a day.

TYPES OF HEARING LOSS

We usually define hearing loss as either sensorineural or conductive. It's useful to understand the difference since it will help explain what is normal and what is not.

Sensorineural hearing loss involves the inner ear, cochlea, or the auditory nerve. Causes of sensorineural hearing loss can include thyroid problems, multiple sclerosis, and autoimmune disease. This is the type of hearing loss associated with aging. *Conductive* hearing loss involves any cause that limits the amount of external sounds that gain access to the inner ear. Therefore, it's mainly caused by outer ear and middle ear problems. For instance, it occurs when the ear canal is completely closed off, or if the eardrum is perforated, or if the middle ear is filled with fluid. Examples include impacted wax, trauma, psoriasis, middle ear infections, tumors, polyps, and trauma.

Mixed hearing loss, consisting of both types, does exist but is quite rare.

Important Questions

When evaluating hearing loss and trying to decide whether it's a normal part of aging, I ask the following questions:

- When did the hearing loss first start?
- How has it changed over time? Has it gotten better? Has it gotten worse?
- How quickly has it changed—over days, weeks, months, or years?

- How well can you understand spoken words?
- Are you dizzy?
- Do you hear ringing?
- Is the hearing problems only when there is background noise, or do they occur in quiet settings as well?
- Is there any type of drainage from the ear?
- Is there any type of ear pain?

Remember, normal hearing loss due to aging usually starts around our sixties, worsens slowly over time, is not painful, and doesn't cause any type of physical symptoms, such as fluid oozing from the ears.

TESTS FOR HEARING LOSS

Because some degree of hearing loss is common after age 60, and because problems with hearing impact quality of life, I recommend that all patients get their hearing tested at age 60. Testing can be done in a doctor's office as well as at specialty clinics.

Unfortunately, many doctors do not routinely test for hearing loss. Can you remember the last time your doctor used a tuning fork to test your hearing? I hope recently, but the reality is that you've probably never seen a tuning fork. The tuning fork is a simple piece of medical equipment that can help identify a hearing problem and distinguish between the two types of hearing loss.

I use a tuning fork to perform two tests: Rinne and Weber.

For the *Rinne* test, the tuning fork is placed on the mastoid bone behind the ear and compared to when the tuning fork is just placed in front of the ear, then manipulated so that it makes a sound. The test is normal when the sound is louder when next to the ear versus next to the bone. An abnormal test usually means there's some type of conductive hearing loss.

For the *Weber* test, the tuning fork is pressed on the middle of the forehead. Then the person is asked if he or she hears the sound louder in one ear. Since the fork is in the middle of the forehead, the sound should be the same in both ears—if the patient has normal hearing, or if the person has the same exact hearing loss in both ears. If a person is already complaining of hearing loss and the sound is louder in the "good" ear, the problem is likely a sensorineural hearing loss. If the sound is louder in the "bad" ear, the problem is likely conductive.

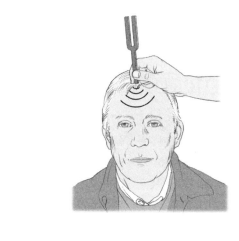

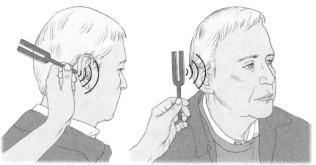

Weber and Rinne Hearing Tests—As discussed, the Weber hearing test *(top)* and Rinne hearing test *(bottom)* use a musical tuning fork to help diagnose certain types of hearing loss in an unhealthy ear.

Hearing: What's Normal and Not Normal As We Age

Normal	Not Normal
Difficulty hearing the television or conversations after age 60	Sudden hearing loss
Ear pain on plane rides	Ear pain during a typical day
Buildup of earwax	Oozing discharge
Infrequent ringing in ear	Frequent ringing in ear with dizziness

I mention these terms because when a person has a sensorineural hearing loss on only one side, the next step is typically a CT scan or an MRI. This is because we need to make sure there's not a more serious condition causing the hearing loss.

There's another test you can administer at home to check your hearing; it's called the whispered voice test. To perform it on someone else, have the person stand about an arm's length behind you, with their back turned toward you. They close off one ear with their finger while you turn and whisper some words or numbers in their other ear. Ask the person to repeat what they heard you say, and then repeat this test with the other ear. Then you can switch sides and let the person perform this test on you. Believe it or not, this is actually a pretty good way to diagnose hearing loss. Try it today, and if the person (or you) has trouble repeating what was whispered in his or her ear, that person should see a doctor for additional tests.

When I detect hearing loss in a patient, I order some general labwork to rule out possible underlying conditions such as diabetes. Thyroid tests can also determine if hyper- or hypothyroidism is causing hearing loss. Finally, syphilis still exists, and even if one was affected a long time ago, hearing loss can occur much later in life.

MEDICATIONS THAT CAUSE HEARING LOSS

People are often unaware that medications can cause hearing loss. The most common medication that can harm the ear is antibiotics. These include vancomycin, erythromycin, tetracycline, gentamicin, amikacin, neomycin, and tobramycin. Cancer drugs such as cisplatin and flurouracil can also cause hearing loss. Loop diuretics and even Viagra have been associated with hearing loss. By no means am I suggesting that you will develop hearing problems if you take these drugs. However, you should be aware of the possibility—even though it is low—that these drugs can affect your hearing. So if you do develop some hearing problems while you're on these drugs, you need to mention it to your doctor, who will probably change your prescription.

WAX IN THE EARS

The fancy medical term is *impacted cerumen*. We all get wax in our ears. And trying to get wax out of the ear with cotton swabs does not work. So stop trying to dig wax out of the ears—I've seen several patients with perforated eardrums due to overly aggressive earwax removal. I even had a patient who developed paralysis of his facial muscles by perforating his eardrum with a cotton swab. So be gentle with those ear canals!

I have to admit there is great satisfaction when removing earwax. I've had at least 25 patients over the years who have come in complaining of hearing loss in one ear (remember—that's not normal in one ear!). On the exam, there's a glob of wax preventing me from seeing anything. After softening the wax and flushing it out with water, gobs of wax are removed . . . and . . . miracle . . . the patient can hear again! It may not be Lazarus rising from the dead, but it's still pretty gratifying to give back someone's hearing!

Most wax dissolves on its own. If you do have a large amount of wax that is bothering you (oozing, itching, or affecting sound), see your doctor or purchase an earwax removal kit from your local pharmacy. They're cheap, safe, and effective.

EAR INFECTIONS

Ear infections are common in kids as well as adults. They almost always occur in the middle ear, and we call it *otitis media*. Nearly 90 percent of school-aged kids develop an ear infection at some point. Ear infections are kind of like pinkeye; everyone seems to get it at some point in his or her life, typically more than once. The infection often causes fluid to accumulate in the ear. Since it is an enclosed space, the ear does not tolerate fluid well. That causes pain, a sense of fullness, and hearing loss. All of those symptoms should make you suspect infection. When we treat the infection, the symptoms typically disappear.

POPPING

If you've been on a plane or driven through the mountains, I'm sure you've experienced "popping" in your ears. It is normal for your ears to "pop" when your body experiences a change in cabin pressure. Basically, when we go up or down in altitude, the pressure outside the ears becomes different from the pressure inside our ears. That difference in pressure can actually change the shape of your eardrum briefly, causing pain.

To prevent the temporary discomfort of "popping," you have to make the pressure equal on both sides. Swallowing forcefully or chewing gum often does the trick. It basically opens up the eustachian tube, which connects the throat to the middle ear, getting rid of the pressure difference. I point this out because it's actually the opening of the eustachian tube that causes the "pop" we hear. It's not your eardrums bursting, as many people often worry!

RINGING IN THE EARS

Yep, there's a medical term for that—it's called *tinnitus*. You hear ringing in your ears or perhaps "humming," "whistling," or sometimes "buzzing"; it would be normal if others heard it, but no one else can. It usually comes and goes; it rarely lasts all the time. Tinnitus needs to be evaluated by a doctor. There are many reasons one can develop tinnitus; some are serious, some are not. It can be part of normal hearing loss associated with aging, but don't automatically assume that unless you have a complete workup and exclude other causes. Too often, we simply say "that's because you're getting old," which is simply not true.

HEARING LOSS WITH DIZZINESS

Dizziness is never considered normal. There are many reasons people can get dizzy, but dizziness combined with hearing loss always needs to be examined thoroughly. Two conditions to be aware of come to mind.

The first is *Ménière's disease*. Ménière's disease is a disorder of the inner ear that results in hearing loss (usually just on one side), tinnitus, and dizziness. The key distinction is the dizziness associated with Ménière's often lasts for hours. The person typically says the room is spinning, although sometimes she says she feels like she's spinning while the room stays still. The symptoms often get worse with movement, even just walking around. The dizziness, however, is not constant; it does not last all day. If that's the case, you don't have Ménière's.

In the early stages of Ménière's, hearing loss usually occurs in

FIVE TIPS TO PRESERVE HEARING

1 Do not listen to loud music, and don't let your children blast music in their earpieces. Don't put any sound-emitting device at a volume more than half of what's permitted. What does this mean? If the volume level goes up to 10, don't exceed 5. Your ears will thank you!

2 Invest in a pair of noise-reduction headphones. They can be a bit expensive, but they're worth it. Be sure to wear them when you're around loud noise. Once your hearing is damaged, it's permanent. Prevention truly is key. Earplugs, though less effective, can also help.

3 Do not place anything smaller than your elbow into your ear canal.

4 Get a hearing exam if you are experiencing hearing problems or every 3 years after you turn 60.

5 If you develop age-related hearing loss, get and use a hearing aid.

the low tones and fluctuates. As the disease progresses, hearing loss becomes more severe and ultimately permanent. Ménière's disease can sometimes be treated with medicine but typically requires surgery.

Acoustic neuroma is another serious condition that can cause mild dizziness, hearing loss, and ringing in the ears. It's a tumor of the eighth cranial nerve—that's the nerve that connects the ear to the brain. Even though it is a tumor, it is not cancerous and cannot spread anywhere. Acoustic neuromas almost never impact anyone before the age of 35, so it's not likely the cause of symptoms if you're at least approaching your forties. It's also pretty rare, affecting fewer than 5,000 people a year. Still, you want to be on the lookout for it. Untreated, it can actually cause your brain to compress, which is dangerous. If you suspect an acoustic neuroma, see your doctor for an MRI. Treatment is surgery, though it's important to note that surgery is not always 100 percent effective and may result in permanent hearing loss.

IMPROVING HEARING

Don't underestimate the importance of hearing in our lives. I have seen quality of life decrease significantly in patients who have hearing loss. Hearing problems often cause low self-esteem, and that can lead to social withdrawal. Because people are embarrassed by their hearing problems (especially problems hearing conversations), they often don't go out as much and become isolated.

Case Study

Jackie is a 54-year-old business executive. Other than high blood pressure, she is in pretty good health. She reads a lot of women's health magazines and surfs the Web for tips on keeping healthy. At a recent visit, she complained of some decreased hearing and a feeling of fullness in one ear after a cross-country flight. "I feel like my ear didn't pop right on the plane," she said. I examined both ears and noticed that she had a large amount of wax in her left ear. We put some softener in there, and she came back the next day to irrigate the ear. A fair amount of wax came out, and she said that she could hear better, although it still didn't feel quite right.

Jackie came back 2 weeks later and said her symptoms had returned, and she hadn't traveled since her last visit. "I meant to tell you last time that I've also had some ringing in my ears for the past few months. It's not all the time, and it's worse at night." I used my tuning fork to perform the Weber and Rinne tests. They were not normal.

I decided to order an MRI of Jackie's brain. As I suspected, it showed an acoustic neuroma. Surgery was scheduled within 2 weeks and was successful. Today, Jackie is doing quite well. The dizziness and ringing in her ears are completely gone. Her hearing is not completely restored, but it's about 90 percent better.

This can make them depressed and, some scientists believe, can even accelerate dementia.

The good news is that hearing aids do benefit people with age-related hearing loss. They may even help those people who have ringing in their ears. They do not, however, restore normal hearing. They work primarily by making sounds louder.

The problem is that many people do not want to use a hearing aid because of cosmetic issues—they don't want to appear to be disabled—or because they don't like how sound is transmitted through the device. As a result, fewer than one out of five adults with significant hearing loss utilizes a hearing aid. Of those who do purchase one, fewer than half regularly use it. This is a big mistake. Modern hearing aids are small, sometimes barely noticeable, and huge improvements have been made in the quality of their transmission, allowing people to make adjustments in the sound volume so that they can hear different frequencies.

Some patients have asked me about cochlear implants. Cochlear implants are devices that are used to provide a sense of sound to people who are either deaf or severely hard of hearing. They consist of two pieces; one is behind the ear, while the other is under the skin. These implants are not hearing aids. While hearing aids mostly make sounds louder, cochlear implants actually bypass the damaged portions of the ear and stimulate nerves, which then send signals to the brain. It's physics at its finest!

Like hearing aids, implants do not restore normal hearing. A big drawback is that hearing through a cochlear implant is not the same as normal hearing. It actually takes time to relearn how sound is transmitted to the brain. However, if people are willing to spend the time to learn how to use them, they vastly improve quality of life.

Answers to true/false statements: False, True, False, True, False

Chapter 8

SNOOZE or LOSE

True or False

As we get older, we need less sleep. _____

As we get older, we need more sleep. _____

Once you get past 80, you don't dream. _____

Napping during the day is typical and to be expected as we get older. _____

(Answers at the end of chapter)

I'm not going to sugarcoat it: The way you experience sleep is going to change as you age. To help you understand what is normal and what is not normal, let's review a little bit about sleep.

I know, you're thinking, "It's just sleep. I do it every day. How complicated can it be?" But despite what you may think, sleep is actually one of the body's most complicated processes. At the simplest level, sleep is a state where the mind and body seem to enter a "rest mode," allowing most external stimuli to be blocked from your senses. Did you know that your body temperature actually decreases by a degree or two when you sleep? Your blood pressure also can drop a little (but no, sleep is not an effective strategy to lower your blood pressure!), and your breathing even slows down. Contrary to popular belief, your brain doesn't actually shut down, but remains active. It just enters a different type of mode. Think of it as being like the "sleep mode" of your laptop.

Some of you might believe that the brain isn't doing anything useful while we're out, and therefore you don't think sleep is important, but you're wrong. Medical science cannot yet fully explain sleep, but increasingly sophisticated technologies are beginning to shed some light on the importance of our sleep. For example, through EEG and MRI imaging, we can observe changes in the brain's function throughout the stages of sleep. Sleep is not merely "rest" but a time when important processes, such as cell repair, are carried out.

Sleep is divided into several stages:

Stage 1. This represents light sleep with slowly rolling eye movements. You might notice a sudden limb movement during this stage. You might experience this on a crowded, uncomfortable plane, at a boring lecture, or snoozing in front of the television. You start to fall asleep, have a limb jerk, and then wake up!

Stage 2. During this stage, eye movements decrease or muscle tone is reduced.

Stage 3. Along with stage 4, this is considered slow wave sleep, or deep sleep. Deep sleep has no eye movements or involuntary muscle contractions or movements.

Stage 4. During this stage, it is hard to arouse someone. You were probably in this stage if someone had to shake you to awaken you. Or maybe a grandchild had to shout in your ear to wake you up early one morning, and it took you a while to orient yourself to where you were.

Rapid eye movement (REM). This is one of the most important stages, and it's where dreaming occurs.

I'm afraid these terms are not very creative. Certainly "Stage 3" lacks something of the flair of, say, "Mid-Level Dream State Slumber," which is how some scientists refer to it. However, the terms

do serve the purpose for which they are intended, which is to out-
line the basic levels we go through as we sleep. And if you understand how those stages of sleep change as we age, it will help
explain what is normal and what isn't.

When I discuss sleep with patients, I always distinguish
between REM and non-REM (Stages 1 through 4). From the time
you go to bed until you wake up, there are quite a few things going
on (that's why I referred to sleep as complicated!). Your body actually alternates between REM and non-REM sleep throughout the
night. Unfortunately, it's not an orderly process. But I will try to
present it in as organized a fashion as I can.

As you get into bed and close your eyes, Stage 1 begins. After
a few minutes, sleep follows. It is normal to take anywhere from
30 to 40 minutes to cycle through Stage 2 through 4. This is where
it gets a little confusing. You can then go through Stage 3, then
back to Stage 2, and finally into REM sleep. In other words, you
don't progress in a nice linear fashion, meaning Stage 1 to Stage 2
to Stage 3 to Stage 4 to REM. Rather, you go back and forth
between the stages. This matters because REM sleep is fairly different from the other four stages. For instance, during REM sleep,
your heart rate and breathing actually can increase; your muscle
tone, however, decreases dramatically, so there is little body movement. A person is usually in REM sleep when others remark how
peaceful he or she looks while sleeping.

But don't be fooled by this lack of physical motion. Although
your body is not moving, your brain is actually quite active during
REM sleep. As I mentioned earlier, it is during REM sleep that we
dream. You won't dream if you don't enter REM sleep. Non-REM
and REM sleep alternate in 90- to 110-minute cycles throughout the
night. A normal sleep pattern has three to five cycles. That's why
you often have several different dreams, even if you can't remember
all of them.

Several different areas of the brain affect sleep, although the alternation of the states of being asleep and awake is largely regulated by the hypothalamus, the part of the brain that links the nervous system to the endocrine system (a system of glands, each of which secretes a type of hormone to regulate the body). Drugs or conditions that affect the hypothalamus will affect your sleep cycle.

As we age, we experience the following changes in our sleep cycles:

- Increased Stage 1
- Decreased Stages 3 and 4
- Decreased REM

What does this mean? Because of these changes in the stages, when we get older, the quality of our sleep decreases. Our sleep often becomes less efficient—meaning we have less deep sleep (Stages 3 and 4) and more time is spent in lighter sleep. You've probably noticed this already. You are more sensitive than you used to be to environmental variables such as noise, light, and temperature changes. As a result, you awaken more often. This translates to more difficulty in maintaining sleep throughout the night. Sleep often becomes fragmented. It is not like when we were teenagers and could fall asleep anywhere, anytime, and not wake up again until our parents made us get up for school. You may also have noticed that either you seem to have fewer dreams than you once did or you have trouble remembering them as easily as you did when you were younger. That's because we dream during REM sleep, and with a decrease in REM sleep, we dream less.

In recent years, we've learned a wealth of new information about sleep and aging. What is particularly interesting is that most of the changes to our sleep cycles actually occur throughout our twenties to sixties. We just don't notice them as easily

Case Study

Patsy is a 70-year-old widow who was brought in to see me by her daughter, with whom she currently lives. Patsy's daughter was concerned that her mother seemed to be sleeping more during the day and also seemed to be groggy in the morning. She also told me that her mother seemed less interested in her usual activities.

Patsy admitted that she's been sad since the death of her husband about 2 years ago, but otherwise feels okay. She is being treated for high blood pressure and high cholesterol, though she said that sometimes she forgets to take her medicine. She said that she argues with her daughter over the temperature of her bedroom; she typically thinks it is too cold, while her daughter says it is too hot. Otherwise, she said that she basically feels the same as she has for years.

The physical portion of her exam was largely normal, except for a resting heart rate in the 50s. Her basic lab tests, including a chemistry profile and cell count, were normal. She did screen positive on a depression test. I started her on an antidepressant, offered counseling (which she declined), and asked to see her again in 3 months. Patsy missed that appointment but did return in 6 months. At that time, she said she felt

because the changes are often subtle and happen over decades. So when I noted that Stage 1 increases, this translates to only about 5 to 10 more minutes to actually fall asleep. As we go through the forties and fifties, we do wake up more often after having fallen asleep, but these awakenings typically last less than a minute. Again, these are small changes, but you should be aware of them. After age 60, it's not normal for our sleep patterns to change much at all.

Here's the critical point: Normal aging is associated with small reductions in total sleep time, maintaining sleep, deep sleep, and dreaming. It does not significantly impact the ability or time it takes to fall asleep, nor does it change the total amount

the same—"no difference." She did say she was taking her medication. I adjusted the dose and saw her again in 3 more months. She showed up on time, and again said nothing had changed. She was still sleeping more often than usual, still feeling sad, still lethargic, and still fighting with her daughter over the thermostat in the house!

Something just didn't seem right to me. So I ordered some more tests, including one for her thyroid. Her tests came back with a high TSH and low free T4. This meant she was hypothyroid; she had an underactive thyroid gland. (There is a reverse feedback mechanism for the thyroid, so if TSH is high, the thyroid hormones are typically low.) Patients who are hypothyroid often show fatigue, lethargy, muscle weakness, dry skin, weight gain, and temperature intolerance, especially to the cold. These symptoms can sometimes be hard to tie together, so hypothyroidism often is overlooked. I started Patsy on Synthroid, and after some adjustments to her dose, within 6 months, she was much more engaged with her daughter and family. More importantly, she was sleeping 7 hours a night, with only a few awakenings. She eliminated any daytime naps.

of sleep time we need. Rather than a consequence of aging, poor sleep as we get older appears to be an indicator of health status. If you are not sleeping well or if an elderly parent is not sleeping well, it's not because you or your parent is getting old—it's usually a

Sleep: What's Normal and Not Normal As We Age

Normal	Not Normal
Lighter sleep	Routine daytime naps
Awake more often	Sleep more than 10 hours
Fewer dreams	Sleep less than 6 hours
Sleepwalking	Difficulty in falling asleep

sign of an underlying health problem or a side effect of the medications used to treat those problems. Most older adults who are healthy rarely have sleep problems.

As mentioned, trouble falling asleep is not a normal part of aging. How do you define "trouble"? It should not take more than 10 to 15 minutes to fall asleep at night. *Insomnia* is typically defined as being unable to obtain restful sleep or enough sleep. We classify types of insomnia based on duration: *Transient insomnia* lasts up to several days; *short-term insomnia* may last up to 3 weeks; and *chronic insomnia* is a condition that persists for more than 3 weeks. All of us will experience a few instances of difficulty falling asleep and maintaining sleep in our lives. Who hasn't experienced a sleepless night worrying about finances, a job, a relationship, or the health of a loved one? However, if you are having trouble falling asleep on a regular basis (several nights a week or even a few times a month), you should see a doctor.

I mentioned earlier that as we get older, we have lighter sleep, so we awaken more often. But remember, these awakenings last less than a minute, and typically do not occur more than three times a night.

DAYTIME NAPS

Increased daytime drowsiness is not a normal part of aging. So if you or your elderly parent is sleeping quite a bit during the day, talk with a doctor. Such daytime drowsiness is often due to medical conditions such as *sleep apnea,* which prevents you from getting restful sleep at night, resulting in daytime fatigue. Sleep apnea is much more common nowadays largely due to the increase in obesity (no pun intended!). For more on sleep apnea, turn to page 134.

Depression is another condition that can be responsible for sleep loss. Depression is common in the elderly, especially in those who are widowed or live alone. There are some estimates that nearly 40 percent of those persons suffering from insomnia have major depression. It often is necessary to treat the underlying disease before sleep will improve.

I often see patients or talk with patients' family members who are concerned about daytime napping. Quite frankly, some of this desire to sleep during the day grows from boredom. Many folks retire and simply don't have enough to keep them as busy as they once were. Too often, as we age, we either plop ourselves in front of the television or caregivers place dependent elderly parents in front of the television while they take care of other tasks. What do many people do when they sit in front of the television? That's right—they close their eyes and go to sleep. So sometimes daytime napping is due to our own making. That's one more reason to have hobbies and maintain personal interaction as we age through the decades.

Our elderly parents do not normally need naps during the day; they do not revert to the sleep needs of infancy. I know many of us think we are helping our loved ones out, or even in our own circumstances, conserving energy by napping during the day, but there is no medical or physiological reason to nap during the day as an older adult.

Unpredictable sleep habits, such as being unable to stay awake while engaged in a conversation, are also situations that warrant medical investigation.

HOW MUCH SLEEP IS ENOUGH?

You do not need more sleep as you age. Nor do you need less sleep. The quantity of sleep you need as you age should be about the same as when you were younger—approximately 7 to 8 hours.

Too little sleep is unquestionably bad for your health. It can cause a heart attack, lead to weight gain, increase your risk of cancer, and even increase your chances of dying prematurely. But what about the flip side: Is it possible to get too much sleep? And what counts as "too much"?

A recent study published in the *Journal of Sleep Research* looked at the association between the amount of time we spend sleeping and our overall health. After reviewing the results from more than 20 other studies, researchers discovered that adults who sleep more than 9 hours per night on average experienced more health problems, such as obesity and stroke, than those who got a restful 7 to 8 hours. Some scientists believe that too much sleep is actually *more* dangerous to our health than too little sleep.

I'm not talking about those of us who try to "catch up" on sleep on the weekends, hoping to make up for the nights we sleep too little. (I might point out, however, that there's no such thing as "catching up on sleep"—more on that later.) The exact mechanism for the increased health risks associated with too much sleep is not known, but some think longer sleep leads to less exposure to daylight, as well as lower levels of beneficial stress. That's right: Some stress can be beneficial. Experiencing a mild level of stress can create a burst of energy that gives us the ability to get more tasks done, and it can help keep us alert in important situations.

The misconception that older folks need more sleep seems to stem from the fact that we undergo a time shift as we get older. Some elements of our biological clocks, and changes to our circadian rhythms, shift to earlier bedtimes and wake-up times. But our environment also plays a role in this shift. Take, for example, the fact that many people seem to think that once retired, they should start eating dinner at 5:00 p.m. (sometimes even 4:00 or 4:30 p.m. for the early birds!), and move their bedtime forward to 9:00 p.m. If our elderly parents are eating dinner at 5:00 and turn out the lights by 9:00, is it any wonder they're up by 6:00 a.m. every day? If you're going to bed at 9:00 p.m., you don't need to sleep to 8:00 in the morning the following day. It's too much sleep! So if you find yourself or your older loved ones spending more than 8 hours asleep, it's time to make an appointment to see a doctor.

Like most people, I do like a good night's sleep. One of the reasons I did not go into surgery or anesthesiology is that I don't like to get up before 6:00 a.m.! I also recognize that developing a good sleep regimen is important for good health. So like many others have probably told you, I encourage you to try to establish a regular sleep time in the evening and wake-up time in the morning and stick with it every day, including weekends. Sleeping longer on weekends actually messes up our biological clocks. It's only natural that there are going to be days when you sometimes get more, and sometimes get less sleep. But aim for 7 to 8 hours of sleep a night for optimal health. Like a lot of things, too much sleep isn't good for you!

SLEEPWALKING

We often joke about sleepwalking, but it's a real condition. You may have heard about people who get up in the middle of the night and wander down to the refrigerator, eat a whole meal, and go back to bed. It sounds like a convenient excuse for weight gain, but it can really happen! Scientists aren't sure exactly why sleepwalking occurs. In the past, doctors thought it was related to epilepsy, psychosis, or even hysteria. Remember the stages of sleep? Well, sleepwalking occurs during Stages 3 and 4. It's during these stages that the body can still be active at a slow pace, while the brain is sleepy. It's almost a type of transition—the person is not fully awake, but not fully asleep. Sleepwalking is much more common in adolescents than in adults. Typically, it doesn't cause significant problems.

It is important to distinguish sleepwalking from a condition that often occurs in the elderly and is not normal. This condition is called *sun downing*, and the person often gets up at night and wanders around the house. This is a dangerous condition that should always be evaluated by a doctor, especially if it is associated with some confusion. Sun downing is sometimes the result of medication side effects, or it may indicate early-onset dementia.

SNORING AND SLEEP APNEA

If you or your spouse snores, you know well that many a marriage has struggled over a snorer. Snoring can be a common condition, but it is not part of the normal sleep process. Snoring is caused by vibrations against the wall of the throat (the soft palate, to be more precise). Basically, the tongue falls back in the throat; if there is loose muscle tone or weak muscle, the wall of the throat starts to collapse. Imagine if air was passing through a tube and you squeezed on the tube—it would start making a squeaking noise. The throat wall collapsing causes the harsh, loud, snorting, choking noises associated with snoring.

Snoring can occur at any age, but it doesn't usually start to occur regularly until we are in our forties. Excess weight increases your likelihood of snoring, as excess weight puts extra pressure on the chest and throat, reducing the size of your airways. Snoring is also more common in men than women. Nearly a third of adults will snore at some point in their lives.

Many people dismiss snoring as just a normal part of the aging process, but it is not. If you or your partner snores several times a week, it's not normal, and you should see your doctor. You might even need to have a sleep study.

Although it seems like the person who's snoring is resting comfortably, he is not. (Though they never seem to be woken up by their own snoring, do they?) Snoring interrupts the sleep cycle, which means that people who snore don't spend as much time in deep sleep (Stages 3 and 4) as they actually need. As a result, snorers often are sleepy during the day, which can cause accidents, memory loss, increased blood pressure, and decreased sex drive. I am most concerned when people stop breathing while they are snoring. So are most of my patients, because that's usually when the spouse or partner marches them into the doctor's office! We call this condition sleep apnea.

Apnea is a Greek word meaning "without breath." People with sleep apnea stop breathing for a few seconds during their sleep until their central nervous systems kick in and "remind" them to take a breath. This typically happens hundreds of times during a night. It's a scary thing for a loved one to witness their spouse or parent literally gasping for air in their sleep. The good news is that the stoppage of breath lasts only a few seconds. The bad news is that sleep apnea is a serious health condition that needs to be treated.

If ignored and left untreated, sleep apnea can increase a person's risk of developing diabetes, heart problems, headaches, and neurological problems. Since people with sleep apnea don't get adequate rest at night, daytime sleepiness is another consequence, and it can decrease job performance as well as increase chances of traffic accidents.

There are effective treatments for both snoring and sleep apnea. Your doctor may ask you to spend the night in a sleep lab so that your sleeping patterns, breathing, and blood pressure can be monitored. If you do have sleep apnea, lifestyle changes including weight loss, use of nose- and mouthpieces, tongue exercises, surgery, and breathing devices such as the CPAP machine can all be effective alone and in combination.

SEVEN TIPS FOR GOOD SLEEP

1 Establish a regular sleep time in the evening and wake-up time in the morning and stick with it every day, including weekends. Sleeping longer on weekends actually interferes with the natural rhythm of our biological clocks. There's no such thing as catching up on sleep.

2 Avoid exercising within an hour of bedtime. Despite the logic that physical activity tires you out and would therefore make you more ready for bed, exercise actually increases your heart rate and releases cortisol, a hormone produced in reaction to stress. As we get older, it takes more time to go back to our resting heart rates. It's hard to fall asleep when our hearts are pumping fast.

3 Do not drink fluids within 2 hours of bedtime. One of the reasons why people get up late at night is to empty their bladders. As we reviewed in Chapter 4, as we get older, our bladder capacity gets smaller. So skip that glass of water on your nightstand before bedtime, and avoid any drinks that contain caffeine in the evening.

4 Insulate your bedroom against loud noise. It does not have to be the "cone of silence" from *Get Smart* episodes (and come to think of it, that never worked!). But since we are more prone to arousal as we age, try to eliminate anything that is likely to startle you. Also keep the room dark. Light serves as a stimulus to our eyes; again, minimize external stimuli.

5 Send the right message to your biological clock. Darkness signals the pineal gland in the brain to produce melatonin, a substance that is

GETTING A GOOD NIGHT'S SLEEP

So now that we know what's normal and what's not normal about sleep, it is vitally important to recognize that as we age, we need good sleep. Failing to sleep well has significant effects on daily life. Insomnia doesn't just make you or a loved one feel tired and grouchy. Loss of sleep can decrease our ability to concentrate,

part of the system that regulates the sleep-wake cycle by chemically causing drowsiness and lowering the body's temperature. So be sure your sleep area is dark, even if you need to put up curtains. Avoid turning on the lights after you've gone to sleep, as this will stop your brain from producing more melatonin that night. Keep a tinted night-light in the bathroom if you tend to go during the night.

6 Keep your bedroom temperature on the cool side. All too often, we get overheated and uncomfortable in bed. How many times have you woken up and had to shed some blankets to fall back asleep? Research suggests that the optimal temperature for sleep is on the cooler side, around 60° to 68°F. A growing number of studies are finding that the temperature of the bedroom plays a role in many cases of chronic insomnia. Researchers have shown, for example, that insomniacs tend to have a warmer core body temperature than normal sleepers just before bed, which leads to heightened arousal and a struggle to fall asleep as the body tries to reset its internal thermostat.

7 Refrain from alcohol. There are some people who still think having a glass of wine or a cocktail will help them fall asleep. They may nod off immediately and enter Stage 1; however, they will have fragmented sleep since alcohol impacts deep sleep and REM sleep. Alcohol is also a diuretic and will likely require you to get up at night to empty your bladder. And the resulting dehydration may leave your throat dry and in need of water. Talk about a vicious cycle!

interfere with judgment, and create problems at home and at work. Compared with people who sleep well, people who don't often get a good night's sleep are less likely to exercise, eat right, engage in leisure activities, and even have sex. More than 11 million people have had a motor vehicle accident or near miss because they were too sleepy to drive safely. Increasing evidence also points to sleep deprivation as a risk factor for chronic illness, including obesity, diabetes, and cardiovascular disease. A good night's sleep really is essential to good health.

Patients and caregivers often ask me about sleep medications. They typically want to know whether I will write a prescription for a sleep aid. Before I discuss any medications to help them sleep, I prefer to discuss medications they may already be taking that could be keeping them from sleeping. Often an existing medication is the culprit for an interrupted sleep cycle. There are numerous medications that impact sleep, including decongestants, antidepressants, antihistamines, some asthma medications such as theophylline and steroids, and even some heart medications such as beta-blockers. Believe it or not, sleeping pills can also make it difficult to sleep. It's important to talk with your doctor about any current medications you're taking before asking for a prescription sleep aid. Sometimes simply changing the time of day that you take your medicine, or changing the prescription, may be the answer you're looking for.

Sleep aids do offer benefit for short-term use, but I discourage patients from using them. Medication can help, but it is not the only choice. Patients sometimes ask me about prescriptions that increase melatonin production, and there is some data to support melatonin as a sleep aid. The theory is that melatonin decreases as we age, and replacing it may help sleep. But again, medication should never be the first option. Behavioral therapy, lifestyle changes, and other nonpharmacological options can help many patients. Remember, problems with sleep as we age are usually due to some underlying medical condition or declining health status. It's important to understand the reason for the difficulty in falling asleep and maintaining sleep, and treat any underlying medical problems. Many people who have difficulty falling asleep or staying asleep through the night head to their medicine cabinets for an over-the-counter remedy, such as one of the common pain relievers followed by the term "PM." I don't recommend taking these nonprescription sleep aids. Just like prescription medications, your body can become dependent on them. Also, medications such as Tylenol PM and Advil PM were not designed to help with sleep; their intended use is for the treatment of pain. If pain is causing sleep problems, treat the pain, not the insomnia.

Pain is a common reason people have difficulty sleeping. We feel that we just have to deal with the aches and pains of old age, but that's not a good idea for numerous reasons. Among them is that it's hard to get a restful night's sleep if you are experiencing pain from a condition such as arthritis or osteoporosis. Be sure to take some type of pain reliever, such as a nonsteroidal anti-inflammatory drug or acetaminophen an hour or two *before* you go to bed, so you can have some pain relief before trying to fall asleep. Lack of pain management is a common reason older people may not sleep well.

Answers to true/false statements: False, False, False, False

Chapter 9

WHAT A PAIN!

True or False

We all will experience pain as we get older. ____

If you are over 80 years old, you are not eligible
for a knee replacement. ____

If you have daily pain, you should be on narcotics. ____

It's common to take over-the-counter pain
relievers on a daily basis to manage aches and pains. ____

(Answers at end of chapter)

Let's face it—everyone experiences pain. We tend to think of pain as something bad, since it causes us discomfort, but it can actually be beneficial. Pain is a signal from our brains that something is wrong and we need to address the problem. As we approach middle age and beyond, we likely will experience more pain than we did when we were younger. After all, our bodies have undergone a lot of wear and tear, and will often need repair. We can also develop chronic conditions that can give us pain.

It's normal to experience some pain as you get older. How much pain is considered normal? It all depends—how much, how often, and where you experience it.

MIND YOUR P'S AND Q'S

In medical school, we're taught to always ask PQRST about pain:

- Position. Where is it located?
- Quality. Is it sharp, dull, throbbing, stabbing, burning, pounding?
- Radiation. Does it go anywhere (down your leg, up your arm, etc.)?
- Severity. How severe is it on a scale of 0 to 10, where 0 is no pain, and 10 is the worst pain of your life?
- Temporal relationship. What's the timing of the pain—e.g., does the pain occur before or after a meal or an activity? What makes it better? What makes it worse?

The answers to these questions will help you and your doctor determine whether the pain you are experiencing is normal or not.

ACUTE VERSUS CHRONIC

There are basically two types of pain: acute and chronic. As its name implies, acute pain is pain that begins suddenly. Think of a stubbed toe, a broken arm, or an upset stomach. Because it is acute, it does not usually last long, and is typically the result of a specific cause or incident. Acute pain usually disappears when the underlying problem goes away. By its very nature, it should not last more than 6 months—if it does, it is considered chronic pain. Some examples of chronic pain can include headaches, back pain, and joint pain. Chronic pain affects nearly one-third of adults over the age of 50.

To understand chronic pain, it's helpful to know a little bit about the pathophysiology of pain.

HOW PAIN WORKS

How our bodies perceive and manage pain is quite elegant. Acute pain is experienced by the body through what is called an excitatory mechanism; the body modulates pain via an inhibitory mechanism regulated by your neurons. When you cut yourself, your nerves send a message to your brain; it's the brain that allows you to feel the sensation of pain. If that connection between your nerves and the brain is broken, you will not feel pain. Chronic pain is the result of either too much excitatory stimulation or not enough inhibitory action. As a result, pain signals stay around.

TREATMENT OPTIONS

Everyone seems to think that drugs are the only way to relieve pain. That's simply not the case. There are a lot of effective non-drug options for pain management. Depending on the cause of pain, there might be a role for physical therapy, occupational therapy, yoga, tai chi, massage, cognitive behavioral therapy, electrical stimulation, or acupuncture. Nerve blocks sometimes play a role in treating pain as well. The age-old remedy of rest also works wonders.

Pain medicines can be very effective in treating pain, both acute and chronic. The first-line medicines are typically over-the-counter medications known as nonsteroidal anti-inflammatory drugs (NSAIDs). Examples include ibuprofen and naproxen, and even aspirin. There are lots of different brand names, and they all basically work in the same way since they are the same class of drug. However, if you don't get a good response from one, that doesn't mean the others won't work for you. What do I mean? Some people get little relief from ibuprofen, but they get good pain relief from naproxen, even though they are both NSAIDs. Acetaminophen (Tylenol), which is not an NSAID, often does the trick as well. Like all medications, these can have side effects, and depending on the type of pain you have, they may not be strong enough.

If you're unable to manage your pain on your own, talk with your doctor about your options. He or she may prescribe a pain killer, a muscle relaxer, or even an antidepressant. Antidepressants are sometimes used to treat chronic pain in people who are not depressed because they help block the transmission of pain signals in the brain. Antiepileptic medications also interrupt these signals in your brain, and in some situations, they might be an option.

Keep in mind that sometimes we need to use multiple treatment options to get pain relief. Honestly, a lot of pain management is trial and error. I know this can be frustrating, but we're still learning how to best treat pain.

I find that patients often do not take pain medications as directed. What do I mean? Often people take too small a dose or space medications out too far. If you are having pain, I do not recommend that you try to "tough it out," as many people do. Toughing it out, or ignoring the pain, is not a good long-term strategy for pain management. When my patients experience pain, I tell them that they can start with a small dose, but they may use up to the maximum dose if needed, especially if it is an over-the-counter medication such as ibuprofen. They should also take it as often as the label allows. Many people take a pain pill once or twice, and if they don't feel it provides the relief they're looking for, they decide the medicine doesn't work. If the medication doesn't seem to be effective at first, try it again. I recommend using a pain medication for at least four or five doses before you decide whether or not it's right for you.

MOST COMMON PAIN AS WE AGE

As we get older, many of us will experience joint pain, typically in our knees or our hips.

This pain is usually the result of normal wear and tear; our joints actually start to deteriorate with the passage of time. We lose cartilage and fluid, and the joint space narrows. As a result, the bones rub against one another, causing pain and stiffness. It's normal to have aches and pains in our joints once we reach our fifties. If it occurs earlier—in your thirties or forties—that's not normal.

The most common cause of joint pain is arthritis. Arthritis is quite common after we reach age 50. In fact, nearly one out of seven of us will develop arthritis (that makes it almost as prevalent as heart disease).

Although many of us will get arthritis, it's a myth that all people develop arthritis as they age. Your genes play a big role in

Case Study

Vanessa is a 70-year-old grandmother who is quite active. She plays bridge twice a week, and enjoys going to her grandchildren's soccer games and ballerina recitals. For the past 10 years, she has been using ibuprofen to manage the osteoarthritis pain in her knees. Over the past 2 years, the pain has been increasing, and she sometimes has to use a cane. "I'm really starting to feel my age," she remarked on a recent visit. I've been adjusting her pain medications over the past 6 months, and have even prescribed several sessions of physical therapy. When I asked her how she felt, she said, "Usually I can handle the pain, but it just seems to be getting worse. I can't get around like I used to. My knees hurt all day and night."

I've talked to Vanessa about knee replacement surgery a couple of times. Her response has always been, "I'm too old for that. Besides, I don't like the idea of surgery." Vanessa is in fairly good health; other than arthritis, I'm treating her for high blood

determining your risk profile; if your mother or father had arthritis, you are more likely to develop it. But there are other factors as well, many of which you can control through a healthy diet and lifestyle. Obesity is one such factor. All that excess weight puts a lot of stress on our joints, causing damage and inflammation. If you've had a broken bone from some type of trauma, you're also more likely to develop arthritis in that joint as you approach middle age. Finally, poor nutrition also plays a role in the development of arthritis. Your joints need important nutrients to stay healthy.

Treatment of arthritis includes pain medications (including cortisone injections) and physical therapy. But for some people, those options may not offer enough relief. When that occurs, joint replacement is an option. Nearly 600,000 people undergo knee replacement surgery each year, and another 200,000 undergo surgery for hip replacements.

pressure and heart disease. She could benefit from losing a few pounds, and her weight is going up as she has become less active with the joint pain.

At her last visit, I told her I could prescribe an opioid like morphine if her pain was continuing to worsen. "I don't want more drugs," she said. I brought up the option of knee replacement surgery again, reassuring her that plenty of people her age benefit from the procedure. I suggested she talk with her friends about it, since I was fairly certain some of them must have had a joint replacement. Several weeks went by, and then I received a phone call from Vanessa. She had spoken to a friend who'd had the surgery, and she was eager to schedule a knee replacement.

Within the month, she had a left total knee replacement. Four months later, she had the other knee replaced. The recovery has been slow and has taken some effort, but Vanessa is now off all pain medications. Her quality of life has improved significantly.

Pain: What's Normal and Not Normal As We Age	
Normal	**Not Normal**
Occasional pain	Daily pain
Arthritis starting around age 50	Arthritis starting around age 30
Morning pain that doesn't keep you in bed past your normal wake time	Pain that prevents you from getting up in the morning
Depression associated with pain	Pain associated with anger

Whether to have knee or hip replacement surgery should be a decision made by you, your doctor, and of course your orthopedic surgeon. All of you play important and distinct roles.

There are many good reasons to have joint replacement. For instance, you will likely benefit from a knee replacement if you are having severe pain that limits your activities of daily living (going up and down stairs, walking, bathing, standing, getting in and out of chairs, lifting housewares), constant swelling that limits your mobility, and severe knee pain even at rest. If you experience any of these issues, I think you should consider a knee replacement.

The hip is another joint that is commonly replaced as we get older. The reasons for a hip replacement are similar to those for the knee. They can include pain that occurs all day, even at night or at rest, and/or pain that limits your ability to walk, lift your legs, or bend over.

The average age of a patient who has a knee replacement is 65; the average age for hip replacements is about the same. Even more surprisingly, there are a significant number of people in their eighties who undergo surgery for a joint replacement. Age itself really should not be a major factor as to whether or not one gets a new joint; instead, pain, disability, and baseline medical conditions are the main factors. I get very frustrated when people think they're

FOUR TIPS TO PREVENT AND MANAGE PAIN

1 Be active! Regular exercise not only helps to build muscle tone and keep your body healthy, but it also releases endorphins, which act as a natural pain reliever in your body.

2 Manage any medical conditions such as diabetes, high blood pressure, and heart disease. Poor health makes us more prone to pain, and can exacerbate pain we already are experiencing.

3 Don't overlook your psychological health. Your mind has a direct impact on your body. Numerous data point out the importance of maintaining our psychological health to maximize our physical health.

4 If you have been prescribed a pain medication by your doctor, be sure to take it as directed. And when you see a doctor because of pain, be sure to tell him or her all of the treatments you have tried previously.

too old for a joint replacement. Why live the last 10 or 15 years of your life in chronic pain? It's never too late to improve the quality of your life. After all, 80 is the new 70!

Joint replacement surgery has been revolutionized in the past few years. The actual procedure is minimally invasive and rather quick nowadays. It's the rehabilitation afterward that takes time. You must be committed to physical therapy for several hours a week for 8 to 12 weeks to gain mobility.

SUPPLEMENTS

Patients often ask me about supplements as well as natural alternatives to surgery or drugs. The supplements that have been most studied for joint pain are glucosamine and chondroitin.

The theory is that these might reduce joint pain by helping the body to make and protect cartilage. If we have more cartilage, or stronger cartilage in our joints, we likely will have less pain.

So what's glucosamine? Glucosamine is a form of glucose that may help the body make cartilage. Chondroitin is a protein molecule that helps make cartilage elastic. Chondroitin is also believed to play a role in preventing our body's enzymes from breaking down cartilage, thereby protecting it and keeping more of it around.

Some studies have shown modest improvement in decreasing pain with taking these two supplements in combination.

SAMe (S-adenosylmethionine) is another supplement that has shown some promise in treating joint pain. It was originally suggested as a natural treatment for depression, but it seems to work better for osteoarthritis. Some studies have shown it is often helpful in reducing joint swelling and improving morning stiffness.

We have known for years that omega-3 fatty acids help lower triglycerides, which then reduces risk of a heart attack. We've recently learned that they may also reduce inflammation in our joints, and thereby reduce pain.

If you're going to try a supplement or natural remedy (after you talk with your doctor), be sure to stick with it for 6 to 8 weeks to see if it helps to relieve your symptoms.

WHAT SHOULD YOU BE DOING NOW TO PREVENT PAIN?

Ideally, the goal is to prevent, delay, or reduce pain. Recent research demonstrates that the body can and does heal itself. That's why it is important to eat a healthy diet and be active. Pain is *not* an inevitable part of aging.

Regular exercise can definitely reduce and delay joint deterioration. Focus on exercises that promote range of motion and strengthen your muscles. In range-of-motion exercises, the focus is on stretching—that's important to help prevent stiffness. Strengthening exercises are my favorite type of exercise, but unfortunately, many people seem to be wary of them. These exercises don't make our joints stronger, but they do make our muscles stronger. Stronger muscles support and stabilize our joints, protecting them from damage. Examples of strengthening exercises include pushups, biceps curls, arm raises, and knee flexions. There are numerous Web sites that offer free instructions on how to perform range-of-motion and strengthening exercises.

Another way to prevent and mitigate pain is to support your body properly when sitting, typing, or otherwise engaged in stationary activities. (Believe it or not, sitting properly cannot only reduce back pain but can also eliminate neck tension and some headaches.) You may be familiar with the term ergonomics. Ergonomics uses medical science and engineering to design furniture and tools that position the body in proper alignment. Understanding ergonomics can help you create a work environment that won't put additional strain on your joints and muscles. When selecting office furniture or supplies, consider your body size and shape, as well as your level of strength and the potential stressors on your muscles and joints. For instance, it matters where you place your computer screen and keyboard in relation to how you sit at your desk. Sometimes you may also need to arrange items on shelves and desks differently. Ergonomic equipment such as chairs that support proper posture, hands-free phones that eliminate neck or back strain, and keyboards that prevent hand and wrist pain can be a little expensive, but I think they are well worth the investment.

Answers to true/false statements: True, False, False, False

Chapter 10

SEX AND ROMANCE

True or False

Many people in their eighties still have sex regularly. _____

Most men become impotent by about age 70. _____

Most women lose interest in sex after menopause. _____

Sexually transmitted diseases are rare
in people over 60. _____

(Answers at end of chapter)

I remember the first time I had to ask an older woman about her sex life. I was still in medical school, and I had to evaluate a new patient and give her a basic physical. As part of the routine checkup, I was supposed to ask if she was sexually active. Here was this gray-haired lady who could have been my grandmother. Like most medical students, I'd never really thought about older adults being sexually active. The whole situation just made me uncomfortable.

I've come a long way since my days as a nervous resident. Now I've talked to 70-year-old women about sex toys. I've listened to men in their eighties who were concerned about the quality of their erections. And I'm aware that even in nursing homes, a lot of sexual activity takes place.

150

Since for most people sex is such a private subject, many people are embarrassed to ask their doctors about any sexual problems they may experience or even ask simple questions to get information that could help to improve their quality of life. Let's take the embarrassment and the mystery out of sex and look at it from a clinical point of view.

THE BASICS

Let's start with the basics: arousal. For a man, being aroused means having an erection. How does the body achieve an erection? The penis contains nerves, muscles, and blood vessels just like the rest of the body. It also contains two long cylinders of spongelike tissue that inflate with blood when a man becomes sexually excited. As the cylinders fill up, the penis becomes erect. The penis becomes soft again when that blood flows back out. For an erection to happen, nerves, blood vessels, and certain hormones all need to work together.

How does a woman's body respond to sexual arousal? Bloodflow to the vagina increases; the labia and outermost part of the vagina swell; and the labia take on a darker red color. Blood flows into the clitoris and, through a mechanism similar to that of the penis, causes it to become swollen and firm. Changes in blood vessels around the vagina allow fluid to leave the blood and act as lubrication on the outside of the vaginal wall. Just like in male arousal, female sexual arousal is the result of a delicate symphony of blood vessels, hormones, and nerves working in concert. In order for arousal to be achieved in either gender, many different body processes are involved; if one system doesn't operate perfectly, problems can occur that interfere with our sex lives.

SEX AND AGING

It's normal to notice changes in your sexual responses as you age.

Physical Changes for Women

Many of my female patients over the age of 45 are concerned about vaginal dryness, which can make sex less comfortable. As estrogen levels decline with menopause, vaginal tissues atrophy, or thin, and are less able to produce lubrication. The vagina can also become narrower, shorter, and less elastic with age. When atrophy of the vulvar and vaginal tissues leads to symptoms, we call it *atrophic vaginitis* or *atrophic vulvovaginitis*. Some women also experience vaginal irritation even when they're not having sex, such as itching or burning. When one of my female patients complains to me about these symptoms, I recommend using a lubricant to make sexual intercourse more comfortable, or using a vaginal moisturizer to ease day-to-day discomfort.

Physical Changes for Men

The issues I hear most often from men in regards to their sexual health concern changes in their erections. As we get older, it's normal for spontaneous erections to happen less often than when we were younger. It's also normal to need more stimulation than you may have needed in the past to achieve an erection.

You'll see some other differences as the years go by. You probably won't wake up with an erection as often as you used to. Your ejaculations may not seem as powerful as they did 10 or 20 years ago, and they might not produce as much semen. Aging also affects the quality of your erections, which typically aren't as full as they used to be, and don't last as long. You might also need more time to "recover" after a sexual encounter before you can achieve another erection. These changes are all a normal part of the aging process.

COMMON PROBLEMS

Because we tend to keep our sex lives private, there are a lot of things that people assume are normal even though they're not. It takes my patients a long time to work up the nerve to ask me questions about sex. Often, I'm on my way out of the examining room when they say, "By the way, Dr. Whyte . . ." To help you start that conversation with your doctor, here are some of the topics that come up often in my exam room—plus some information about what you can do about them.

Loss of Interest

Some people do experience a diminished sex drive as they get older. For women, declining libido usually occurs around the time of menopause.

I ask a lot of questions when I hear that someone is having problems with desire, because there are so many reasons why desire could disappear. For a woman, it could be the result of vaginal changes associated with menopause—she's having pain with intercourse, or simply doesn't enjoy it as much as she used to. A man might be embarrassed about erectile dysfunction (ED) and avoids having sex with his wife. In these cases, when the physical problem is addressed, desire usually returns.

Sometimes lack of desire has emotional roots; oftentimes when something changes in a relationship and emotional intimacy suffers, physical intimacy is also affected. The major life changes that come with age—such as retirement, health problems, and money issues—can all add stress to a relationship and cause couples to become less connected.

Medications can also affect your sex drive. Antidepressants and opioid painkillers (such as morphine or oxycodone) are known to affect libido. If you're experiencing a loss of desire, you might need to talk with your doctor about the medications you're taking to see if one of them may be contributing to your problem.

The hormonal changes that come with age also affect libido. I'll cover the effects of lowered testosterone levels in men in Chapter 12. For some men, a prescription for testosterone supplements can be helpful. There's also been research that suggests that postmenopausal women with low libido can also benefit from testosterone, but currently there isn't sufficient research for me to recommend this as an option.

Erectile Dysfunction

As mentioned earlier, some degree of erectile dysfunction (ED) is very common as men age. A recent survey of men over the age of 50 found that 37 percent of participants reported difficulty achieving or maintaining an erection. But we also know that ED is linked to certain illnesses that become more common as we age, and that good health can translate into longer-lasting sexual health.

Diabetes is one of the biggest risk factors for ED. People with heart disease, peripheral vascular disease, or stroke are also at higher risk. Smoking can raise your chance of developing ED, too. Other risk factors include high blood pressure, high cholesterol, obesity, and heavy alcohol use. Because of the link with cardiovascular disease, I suggest that all men with ED should see their doctors to be checked for problems such as high blood pressure, high cholesterol, and diabetes.

ED can also be a side effect of certain medications. This includes some blood pressure medicines, antidepressants and other drugs prescribed for mental health, and medications used to treat prostate cancer. Be sure to talk with your doctor about the medications you're currently taking.

And just like declines in desire, ED can also be the result of emotional difficulties. Stressors in your life, problems with your partner, and fears about your health can all affect your erections.

If you suspect that you have ED, the first thing to do is to see your doctor. You can also take some simple steps to improve your health, including:

- Get your cholesterol and blood pressure under control (and your blood sugar, too, if you have diabetes).
- Get plenty of exercise.
- If you need to, lose weight.
- If you smoke, quit.

ED Medications

Most men can also try a prescription pill for ED. The three main options are all in a class of drugs called phosphodiesterase inhibitors. These pills won't turn you into a sex machine, but they can help you have an erection when you want one. All of them work by helping to increase bloodflow to the penis. Some men have to try a couple of different pills to find the one that works best for them.

If your doctor decides you can use a pill, you're most likely to be prescribed one of the following:

- Sildenafil
- Vardenafil
- Tadalafil

Sildenafil can start working in as quickly as 30 minutes; most men will feel its effects within an hour. It generally wears off after about 4 hours, although it may last longer for some men. That doesn't mean you'll have an erection the whole time—just that you've got about 4 hours to carry out your romantic plans. Your body will absorb sildenafil more slowly if you've just eaten a high-fat meal like a burger and fries, which could make it take longer to work. I tell my patients to plan their meals accordingly—maybe go for a healthier option or take sildenafil on an empty stomach. Sildenafil has an interesting side effect: In a small percentage of men, it can cause temporary changes in the way they perceive color. Everything might look bluish, or you might have trouble distinguishing blue from green.

Vardenafil has a chemical structure that's similar to sildenafil, although it's not exactly the same. It also begins working within about an hour and lasts about 4 hours. Like sildenafil, it's best not to eat a high-fat meal before taking it, and it has also been known to cause temporary changes in color vision.

Tadalafil is a pill with a different molecular structure than sildenafil or vardenafil, and as such, it works somewhat differently in the body. This pill's effects can last for up to 36 hours. There is also a lower-dose version available that's meant to be taken every day. The 36-hour dose will start working in about 30 minutes for some men, although it will take longer in others. Men who are just starting the daily dose may have to wait a few days before experiencing the drug's full effect.

There doesn't seem to be one best choice in terms of how well these drugs work. So if you're going to try one, talk with your doctor about the best fit for you in terms of convenience, cost, and safety. Like all medications, ED pills carry certain risks and side effects. For the most part, the potential side effects of each of these drugs are similar. Some men experience headaches or facial flushing; some have reported more serious side effects such as sudden hearing loss or decreased vision. It's not clear if the drugs directly caused those particular problems, but it's something to keep in mind. And you've probably seen the television commercials for ED drugs that warn you to see your doctor if an erection lasts for a specified amount of time. It may seem funny, but the truth is that not only are these long-lasting erections embarrassing and uncomfortable, they can also become dangerous. If the blood doesn't drain on its own, it may need to be drained surgically to prevent permanent damage. It is important to see your doctor if you experience this side effect.

If your doctor recommends an ED drug for you, it's important to talk over your medical history, any medicines you're taking, and even certain lifestyle issues. For example, none of these drugs can be combined with nitrates (such as nitroglycerine for angina), because the combination could cause dangerously low blood pressure. Some recreational drugs contain nitrates, too. And it's a good idea to be careful with alcohol, especially with tadalafil, as it can also cause your blood pressure to drop dangerously low.

Some men ask me if taking ED medication long term could actually make their ED worse—in essence, if taking these drugs will make them "dependent." But taking an ED medication doesn't mean you will always have to take it to get an erection. In fact, a group of researchers studied men who took an ED drug every night for a year, and at the end of that time, had them stop taking the medication. More than half of them had better erectile function than when they started taking the drug. So if your doctor thinks these medications are right for you, there's no reason not to give them a try.

While many men find relief in medications for erectile dysfunction, these prescriptions don't work for everyone. And some men cannot take the pills because of other health problems. If you're in that minority, there are other options. Some men use a medication that's injected directly into the penis or a tablet that's inserted into the urethra. (And yes, some men think about these for about 2 seconds and say, "No way!" But others find that they're able to incorporate one of these treatments into their sex lives and it works just fine for them.) Some have success using a special vacuum device to draw blood into the penis.

If none of these options work, some men choose to have surgery. Your doctor can provide more information on the types of implants that are available.

Sexual Health: What's Normal and Not Normal As We Age

Normal	Not Normal
FOR WOMEN:	
Noticing that your labia and vaginal entrance seem smaller, lighter in color, and drier than they used to	Noticing sores, lumps, or discolored patches
Having pain with intercourse that gets better when you use lubricant, moisturizer, or a local hormone treatment	Having constant vulvar or vaginal pain, itching, or burning
FOR MEN:	
Having less firm erections or erections that don't last as long as they used to	Having erections that don't last long enough for intercourse
Needing more stimulation to have an erection	Having no erections at all
FOR EVERYONE:	
Not feeling as urgent or driven about sex as you used to	Losing your sex drive entirely (although this isn't necessarily a problem, if you're perfectly happy without it)

TESTOSTERONE REPLACEMENT THERAPY

Testosterone replacement therapy is sometimes used to treat erectile dysfunction, but there are still questions about whom it will help and whether long-term use is safe. If your testosterone levels are normal, extra testosterone probably isn't going to solve your ED. If you have low testosterone, though, there's a chance that supplementation might be helpful. You can learn more about this in Chapter 12. If you think low testosterone might be an issue for you, your doctor can give you the latest information and recommendations.

NATURAL ALTERNATIVES

As a general rule, I'm skeptical about "alternative" remedies to treat erectile dysfunction. There are a lot of people out there selling things with no evidence to back them up—no matter what they claim on their Web sites. Some of these substances have been studied for sexual effects in animals but not in people. Some haven't been studied at all. And a few of them do show promise and might be worth a try. Talk with your doctor about any new drug or therapy before you begin use. Here are some of the products that my patients often ask me about:

Yohimbine. Yohimbine is a chemical found in the bark of a tree called yohimbe. You'll find it both as a prescription medicine and at the health food store. A handful of studies in men with ED suggest that it might have a modest effect. If you try it, be cautious of side effects that could include high blood pressure, a rapid heartbeat, anxiety, insomnia, headache, nausea and vomiting, dizziness, and tremors.

L-arginine. L-arginine is a molecule that's found in proteins. Within your body, l-arginine can be transformed into nitric oxide

(NO), which is responsible for an important step in developing an erection. Some fitness enthusiasts use l-arginine as a supplement, believing it allows them to lift more weight in the gym. A few small studies suggest that a daily l-arginine supplement could help some men with ED. L-arginine has the potential to lower blood pressure, so be careful if you're already taking blood pressure medicine. It's not recommended for people who have had a heart attack in the recent past.

Ginseng. Red ginseng, also known as *Panax ginseng,* is thought to promote bloodflow to the penis. Some evidence suggests that ginseng may help with erectile dysfunction. There's a chance that ginseng could lower your blood sugar, so be careful if you're already taking diabetes medicine.

Maca. Maca is an Andean herb that supposedly works as an aphrodisiac. A small study in men with mild ED suggests that it can help with erections.

Ginkgo biloba. Ginkgo may have beneficial effects on blood circulation. It's been studied as a treatment for sexual problems, but so far there's no strong evidence that it works to treat ED.

Horny goat weed. Horny goat weed, also called epimedium (although the first name describes it better, doesn't it?), is sold as a libido booster and sometimes as a treatment for ED. The plant does contain a chemical that appears to act in a way similar to prescription ED drugs, but the effect isn't very strong.

SEXUALLY TRANSMITTED DISEASES

One final word about sex and aging. Actually, two final words: safer sex. Younger adults grew up in the shadow of HIV and AIDS. They're used to the idea of using condoms and getting tested regularly for sexually transmitted diseases (STDs). Not that they always do the right thing, mind you—but it's part of their sexual culture. I find that a lot of single older adults aren't necessarily thinking about STDs when they reenter the dating world, which is a big mistake.

In fact, people over the age of 50 make up 15 percent of new HIV diagnoses.

Condoms can reduce your risk of all sexually transmitted diseases, including AIDS, chlamydia, herpes, gonorrhea, and syphilis. They're not foolproof, though. The safer-sex advice for older adults is the same as for younger ones: Wait until you know you can trust your partner; talk about your sexual histories and risk of STDs; and always practice safe sex. Be aware that drugs and

FIVE TIPS FOR BETTER SEX

1 Don't believe anyone who says old people don't have sex! It's just not true. It's normal and healthy to have sexual feelings well into old age.

2 Invest in a good lubricant. During sexual intercourse, lubricant can help protect vulvar and vaginal tissues that get drier and more delicate with age. If using "lube" is new for you, you can try it out on your own before using it with a partner.

3 Get help for sexual problems. If you're not having erections anymore . . . if your sex drive seems to have disappeared with the years and you want it back . . . if having sex hurts . . . head for your doctor's office. There are lots of things we can do to help.

4 Accept the changes that are normal. Nothing puts a damper on sex like being worried or upset about your body. If you accept the fact that your sexual responses are changing, you can focus on enjoying sex in new ways. Take it slow and figure out what feels good. For some people, sexual intercourse won't be the "main event" anymore, but there are lots of other ways to be intimate with your partner. Different doesn't have to be bad.

5 Practice safe sex. STDs don't care how old you are. Use condoms unless you're in a monogamous relationship with someone you know and trust. And if you do reach that point with a new partner, it's a good idea to both get screened for STDs.

Case Study

Jim is one of my longtime patients. He had been married for 42 years and has been a widower for the past 5 years. When his wife died, I expected Jim would be subject to major lifestyle adjustments. For several years afterward, he had indeed remained somewhat reclusive. During his checkups and wellness exams, we would discuss if he was experiencing depression. Jim made it clear that he was sad at times, but was generally happy and enjoying his life and his beautiful grandchildren. I suggested he get involved in activities at the local Senior Center.

As I was exiting the exam room after his most recent appointment, Jim stopped me with the famous saying, "Oh, by the way, Dr. Whyte . . ." Hesitantly, he expressed his excitement about a woman he's begun dating. He said that things had recently heated up in the relationship, but he was a little nervous about having sex. Jim stated they tried a couple of times this past month, but he could not attain a hard-enough erection. I assured Jim that his anxiety and his condition were normal. We discussed his erectile dysfunction in more detail, and I explained the various treatment options that might improve his erection. He said he would think about it and we could talk more at the next visit.

Two months later, Jim came back for a "walk-in" appointment, and explained he had not experienced any improvements in his erections. "Doc, can I get that pill you mentioned that I see on TV?" he asked. I explained the risks and the benefits of Viagra, and we decided to give it a trial. I instructed Jim on how to properly take the medication and reminded him about the importance of practicing safe sex. One month later he came back in to see me with a sheepish grin, and told me his relationship was back on track.

alcohol can cloud your judgment. Consider asking your potential partner to be screened for STDs—and get tested yourself. And if you use a lubricant with a condom, make sure it's water-based. Oil- or petroleum-based lubricants can cause latex condoms to break.

Answers to true/false statements: **True, False, False, False**

Chapter 11

WOMEN'S HEALTH

True or False

Most women should go on hormone therapy
after menopause. _____

Women don't need to worry about heart
attacks—it's mostly men who have them. _____

Breast cancer screening should start at age 40. _____

Mammography isn't needed after you turn 75. _____

(Answers at end of chapter)

Don't let the title of the chapter fool you—this chapter is not just
for women. In fact, if you're a man, you might learn a thing or two
that will help you care for the women in your life.

As we get older, we all confront some issues that are unique to
our gender. There are certain changes in our health that are a lot
more common in women than in men. In the past, some of these
health issues have been treated as men's concerns even though
they're also vitally important to women's health.

THE DIVIDING LINE

Menopause is a dividing line in a lot of women's lives. Not only
does the menstrual cycle change, but menopause is accompanied

by a number of other changes and health issues. Many women experience hot flashes, sexual changes, and emotional struggles. The risk profile for developing many diseases changes after menopause, too: Women are more likely to have heart attacks, and their risk of developing breast cancer also increases. The rate of bone loss speeds up as well, which puts women at risk of developing osteoporosis. The good news is there's a lot you can do to keep your health on track after menopause. The key is to know what's normal and what isn't.

WHAT'S MENOPAUSE?

Technically, menopause means the permanent cessation of menstruation. That makes it a very specific point in time. When my patients talk about menopause, though, they're usually referring to a much longer process. It can take months or years from the time your menstrual cycle slows down to the time it stops. Doctors call that time period *perimenopause,* or the *menopausal transition.* But even though my gynecologist friends might not like it, I'm going to do what my patients do: I'm going to use the term *menopause* to reference that whole length of time. Once a woman has had her final period, doctors say she's "postmenopausal." I'll use that term to describe the years after the change is over.

The typical age of that final menstrual period is about 51. We don't say menopause is "premature" unless a woman experiences her last period under the age of 40. Most women are postmenopausal by their late fifties.

What happens during menopause is very complicated. Ever since you hit puberty, your ovaries have been making substantial amounts of estrogen. Assuming everything was normal, throughout your adult life they've also been releasing eggs, about one each month, in case you wanted to get pregnant. Every 28 days or so, if you weren't pregnant, the interplay of estrogen and other hormones would lead to a few days of fertility, followed about 2 weeks later by a period.

When you reach menopause, that neat cycle comes to an end. The interplay of hormones begins to change. Eventually, your ovaries stop releasing eggs, and they stop making estrogen and another reproductive hormone called progesterone. And while you won't be aware of all the little changes going on inside your body, it's likely that you'll notice at least some of their effects as you approach menopause. Some women experience a lot of symptoms. Others breeze right through.

How do you know if you might be going through menopause? I've had many female patients make an appointment to come in because they just don't feel right—and they're surprised when I tell them they're experiencing menopause. Here are some common signs and symptoms of menopause:

• **Irregular periods.** Your periods might get longer or shorter. You might skip a few months and think that's it, and then start having periods again. The key is they're becoming irregular. Be careful about birth control during this time, because it may still be possible to get pregnant. I've seen many patients who were shocked that they became pregnant in their forties.

• **Hot flashes.** Many women are curious about what these will feel like—but my female patients tell me, once you have one, you'll know! They describe suddenly feeling warm, sometimes *extremely* warm. They talk about breaking into a sweat and reaching for the nearest magazine or piece of paper to use as a fan. A typical hot flash lasts a few minutes at most, and then things return to normal.

• **Vaginal changes.** As you learned in Chapter 10, estrogen helps keep your vaginal tissue functioning properly. As you go through menopause, that tissue gets thinner, and it doesn't lubricate the way it used to. It's also common to experience some discomfort during intercourse.

• **Urinary tract infections (UTIs).** During menopause, the decline in estrogen may make you more prone to getting UTIs. Why? The level of acidity in your vagina actually changes around the time of menopause, allowing the bacteria that cause infections to grow.

Some women welcome menopause. They're thrilled to be free of the monthly hassle of menstruation, and they're delighted to finally be relieved of birth control measures. Other women dread it. Maybe they haven't had all the children they wanted. Maybe they equate menopause with getting old. Some aren't sure how to feel, and then they worry that they're not having the appropriate reaction. All these feelings are normal.

Around the time you hit menopause, you may begin to experience other symptoms, such as trouble sleeping, irritability, and decrease in libido. These changes may be related to menopause; but oftentimes, they may also be related to other circumstances in your life or underlying health conditions.

If you experience a lot of menopausal symptoms, it might be hard to tell which ones are normal and which ones could be a cause for concern. If you develop any of the following symptoms, it's important to see your doctor. They are not a normal part of menopause.

• **Out-of-control periods.** It's not normal if your periods don't ever seem to end. Really heavy periods or spotting between periods could be signs of a problem, too. So could an unusually short time between periods. Unusual patterns of bleeding sometimes get better on their own after a few cycles, but if they don't, see your doctor. These symptoms may be a sign that you have a uterine polyp or fibroids, both of which are benign growths in your uterus that can be removed. Worst-case scenario, abnormal bleeding could be a sign of uterine cancer.

• **Serious depression.** Many women experience mood swings and some level of irritability during menopause, which is perfectly normal. But if you find that you've become depressed to the point that you can't function normally, or if you feel that emotional instability is interfering with your work or relationships, see your doctor.

• **Internal pelvic pressure.** As you approach middle age, the muscles and other tissues that hold your bladder and uterus in place can weaken. It sounds strange, but your uterus, bladder, or rectum can actually start to protrude into your vagina. This is called *pelvic organ prolapse.* You might see or feel this protrusion—some women say it feels like sitting on a ball. See your doctor if you experience symptoms such as a feeling of fullness or pressure in your lower abdomen, incontinence, or pain during sexual intercourse.

• **Memory loss.** I'm not talking about forgetting where you put your keys or that you promised to pick up the dry cleaning. If you're bothered by symptoms of menopause, it may be hard to keep up your normal level of efficiency. I'm talking about forgetting important things at work, forgetting what you did yesterday, or forgetting what your keys are *for.* If these things are happening, it's time to see your doctor.

HORMONE THERAPY:
THE PROS AND CONS

Hormone replacement therapy (HRT) involves the supplementation of natural or synthetic estrogen and progesterone. When I was in medical school, we routinely prescribed HRT for women who had gone through menopause. The idea was to prevent heart disease and osteoporosis by supplying the body with the hormones that the ovaries no longer produce.

These days, we mainly offer HRT to younger women who are bothered by menopause symptoms such as hot flashes and vaginal changes. But we're cautious. Like many doctors, I use the lowest dose that works for each patient and prescribe treatment for the shortest period of time I can. I also ask each of my patients on HRT to check in with me at least once every 6 months so that we can know when her symptoms seem to be alleviated, and we can take her off the hormones for good.

You may have heard about the link between HRT and health problems, which has gotten a lot of attention in the media. In 2002, a report from the Women's Health Initiative—a 15-year study established by the National Institutes of Health to investigate and address the most common causes of death, disability, and impaired quality of life in postmenopausal women—showed that while hormone therapy could both prevent and improve the symptoms of osteoporosis, it might increase the risk of heart attacks.[1] Further complicating matters, many of the subjects who took part in the study were well past menopause when they started taking hormones, so it's not clear whether or not the risk of heart attack is as great for the younger women who are most often prescribed HRT. So far, it looks like hormone therapy probably doesn't increase the risk of a heart attack in this group. And it might actually decrease the risk of colon cancer.

But there are other risks to consider, and that's why we keep the dose low and aim to stop when the symptoms are over. Hormone therapy raises the risk of blood clots, which can be dangerous if they travel to your lungs. It increases the chance that you'll develop gallbladder disease. It can also raise your risk of breast cancer and stroke. Luckily, these risks are pretty small; the risk of breast cancer increases about 2 percent each year you are on hormone replacement therapy, and the risk of stroke increases by about 1.5 percent. The risk is even smaller if you use hormone therapy for only a short period of time (no more than a couple of years) and are constantly reevaluated. And, to me, there's a big difference between taking a medicine to prevent something that might or might not happen in the future and taking a medicine to treat symptoms that are happening now. Every drug has risks, but it's often worth it to get the benefits.

Most women who choose hormone therapy will receive a combination of estrogen and a type of progestin. If you've had a hysterectomy, you can take just estrogen. The pattern of risks is a little different: For example, in the Women's Health Initiative study, estrogen alone didn't raise the risk of breast cancer or heart attack. There are also different options for receiving hormone therapy, such as taking a pill, applying a gel, or even wearing a patch. Different options will treat different patterns of symptoms.

WHAT ABOUT ALTERNATIVES?

My female patients often ask me about the effectiveness of herbal remedies for menopause symptoms. My general advice is to err on the side of caution. Most of these products do not have rigorous scientific studies to support their use, and if they really worked as well as they claim to, we would have more data to evaluate. Television testimonials are not the measure we use in medicine to determine whether something is safe to put in our bodies!

Black cohosh is a popular herb for treating hot flashes, and a few small studies suggest it might help. Black cohosh seems to be safe, but it has also been linked to a small number of cases of liver disease. I would treat black cohosh like any new supplement or remedy you're considering: Talk with your doctor first. Try it for a few weeks; if you don't see any improvement, throw it away.

A lot of women also ask me about eating more soy, since it contains phytoestrogens, or plant estrogens, that are similar in some ways to human estrogen. Most soy foods are healthy options, though I recommend staying away from highly processed soy products (edamame is a great option). Since soy may work like estrogen, though, it is recommended that women with current or past breast cancer avoid soy foods, as they may promote cancer cell growth.

WOMEN'S BIGGEST FEAR

Even though women are more likely to die from heart disease than from breast cancer (typically more than 300,000 women die from heart disease each year, compared with 40,000 from breast cancer), I find most women's biggest health fear as they age is being diagnosed with breast cancer. As you approach middle age and beyond, your risk of developing breast cancer does increase. That's just a fact of life, so in a way it's normal. But it's important to put that risk into context. Among women who are 60 years old, only 3 out of 100 will be diagnosed with breast cancer in the next 10 years. Within the next 30 years, about 8 in 100 will develop breast cancer.

No one can tell you your exact breast cancer risk. But we are starting to learn about things that influence your risk. Here are some of the risk factors you should be aware of:

• **Age.** About two-thirds of invasive breast cancers are found in women who are 55 or older.

• **Family history.** Your risk approximately doubles if your mother, sister, or daughter had breast cancer. It triples if two close relatives had it. Your risk is especially high if you have a mutation in one of the genes called BRCA1 and BRCA2. Such a gene mutation is often hereditary.

• **Menstrual cycles.** Either starting to menstruate at a young age and/or going through menopause at a late age increases your risk of breast cancer.

• **Pregnancy.** Having many children or having a child at a young age can reduce your risk, although this may not be true for all types of breast cancer.

• **Birth control pills and hormone therapy.** Oral contraceptives slightly increase your risk of breast cancer, though estrogen-progestin contraceptives decrease the risk of endometrial, ovarian, and colon cancers. Using combined hormone therapy (estrogen plus progestin) after menopause also increases your risk of breast cancer.

• **Weight.** Being overweight, especially after menopause, puts you at a higher risk.

As you can see, some of these risk factors are within your control, and others are not. Focus on ones you can control, such as weight management. And if you are at increased risk, be sure to talk with your doctor about having a mammogram.

MAMMOGRAMS AND DETECTION

A 41-year-old female patient recently asked me about having her first mammogram. She didn't have a strong family history of breast cancer, but she sees and hears so much about breast cancer that she thought she should probably get checked out. "I'm so confused, Dr. Whyte," she said. "Last year I heard that it was okay to wait until age 50 to start having mammograms, so I didn't bother. But my best friend's doctor insisted that she have a mammogram the minute she turned 40. I went online to look it up, and I still can't tell what I'm supposed to do!"

You may be confused, too. Should you start at age 40 or 50? Should you go every year, or is every 2 years okay? Is there an age when you should stop?

What you need to understand is that sometimes the experts don't all agree. The truth is that mammograms, like most medical tests, are not perfect, and the experts don't all agree on how often women should get screened. In fact, mammograms are such an imprecise test that even when a mammogram indicates a potential cancer, and you have to have a biopsy, 80 percent of the time the biopsy will come back benign. And even though mammograms do find a lot of actual cancers, sometimes a tumor does not show up or the doctor reading the mammogram misses it.

The younger you are, the harder it is to read your mammogram. Young women have dense breasts, and a mammogram of a dense breast looks kind of like a white blob. It's hard to see what's normal and what's not. As you get older, your breast tissue changes and it becomes easier to see if a tumor is there. Some experts feel that for women under 50, the risk of an unnecessary cancer scare, plus the possibility of missing a tumor even with the test, outweigh the potential benefit. Others feel very strongly that the chance of saving a woman's life makes all the risks worth it.

Many doctors recommend women have a mammogram every 2 years—the idea being that it maintains the benefit of early detection while cutting down on the risk of unnecessary biopsies.[2] But it's also important to know that some types of tumors grow quickly. Talk with your doctor about your specific concerns to determine how often you should have a mammogram.

How long do women need to have mammograms? It really depends on the patient—there's no natural cutoff age. That said, if a woman is elderly and in poor health, a mammogram might not make sense for her. Even if cancer is detected, she might not do well with treatment, and it might not extend her life.

I find that many women consider the risks a small price to pay for the chance to catch a dangerous cancer early. Sit down with your doctor, talk over your family history and your own personal risk of breast cancer, and then decide how frequently you need to get a mammogram. There's no right or wrong decision.

It's important to note that these guidelines are intended for women who are at an average risk. Women at a higher risk—particularly those with a family history of breast cancer—might want to start mammograms at a younger age, be screened more frequently, or have additional tests.

OTHER WAYS TO DETECT BREAST CANCER

Mammograms aren't the only way to screen for breast cancer. Breast exams at the doctor's office may reveal larger tumors. The American Cancer Society recommends a breast exam every 3 years from age 20 to 40 and once a year after that.[3]

Many women with breast cancer find their tumors on their own. If you feel a lump, either by accident or during a self-exam, don't ignore it, even if your last mammogram was normal. Lumps are not considered a normal part of aging and should always be biopsied. Make a doctor's appointment immediately.

Until recently, it was common for doctors to recommend that women examine their breasts once a month to check for cancer. It seemed like every women's organization was handing out instructions, including waterproof reminders you could hang in your shower. Today, don't be surprised if your doctor doesn't mention a self-exam at all.

Why the change? It turned out that telling all women to do self-exams may not actually save lives. If you notice a change in your breast, you should always get it checked out. If you're already doing regular self-exams, or even occasional ones, you don't necessarily have to stop. It may be helpful to know how your breasts normally look and feel, and it's possible you could detect a tumor earlier than you would have otherwise.

If you want to learn to do a self-exam (or make sure you're doing it right), your doctor should be able to teach you. You can't really learn to do this by reading a book. Still, I'll do my best to give you an idea of what a self-exam involves. These instructions are based on a guide from the American Cancer Society. Their breast cancer screening recommendations include self-exam as an option for women—with a health professional's guidance—starting in their twenties.

1. Lie on your back, so your breasts spread out across your chest wall.

2. Put one arm behind your head. This is the side you'll examine first.

3. Using the index, middle, and ring fingers of the opposite hand, make small, overlapping circles over your breast tissue. Repeat each circle three times, using light, medium,

and firm pressure. You're looking for anything that feels different, like a lump that wasn't there before.

4. To keep track of what you've already covered, follow an up-and-down pattern. Start at your armpit and go straight down the side of your chest and then, following imaginary up-and-down lines, work your way over to your sternum. Make sure you go all the way up to your collarbone and down to where you can feel your ribs without any breast tissue over them.

5. Now switch which arm is behind your head, and examine the other breast the same way.

6. Next, stand up and face a mirror. Put your hands on your hips and press down to contract your chest muscles.

7. Look at your breasts. Have there been any changes in size or shape? Does the skin look dimpled anywhere? Any red or scaly spots on your breast or your nipple?

8. Finally, raise one arm up just a little bit and use the fingers of the other hand to examine your underarm. Repeat on the other side.

Here are some other changes to look for, again based on advice from the American Cancer Society.[4] None of these things mean you definitely have cancer—but you should definitely get them checked out.

- A swollen area
- A nipple that has turned inward
- A discharge from your nipple

Even if it's not listed here, if something doesn't look right to you, see your doctor.

WOMEN AND HEART DISEASE

Heart disease is the number one killer of women. On average, men have heart attacks at younger ages than women, but more women than men die of heart disease each year. One reason women are more prone to heart disease than men is because their hearts are typically smaller than men's, which means that their coronary arteries (the blood vessels that feed the heart muscle) are smaller, too. When these smaller blood vessels develop clots or plaques, it can be deadly.

Women over the age of 55 are at the greatest risk of heart disease. Age can also bring on other risk factors such as high blood pressure and high cholesterol. Women tend to die sooner after a heart attack than men, partly because they're often older when a heart attack strikes. If you haven't given it much thought before, menopause can be a useful wake-up call to start paying attention to your heart.

You know what I find very troubling about heart attacks in women? About two-thirds of women who die suddenly from heart disease had never experienced any previous symptoms. That means it's important to do what you can to keep your heart healthy—and also to know how to recognize a heart attack, so you can get help.

The classic symptom of a heart attack is chest pain or pressure. One description I often hear is that it feels "like an elephant is sitting on my chest." It might hurt; it might feel like squeezing; there might be tightness; or it might just be a sense of fullness or discomfort. I like to call it "discomfort" since it can include pain or other feelings. Too many women think that if they aren't experiencing intense pain, they're not having a heart attack. But not all heart attacks cause pain.

Also, chest discomfort is not necessarily the only symptom, and sometimes it's not even the most obvious one. Some other typical symptoms of a heart attack include:

- Pain or discomfort in one or both of your arms, your jaw, your neck, your stomach, or your back—with or without chest pain
- Shortness of breath
- Sweating
- Nausea
- Light-headedness

If something doesn't feel right, asking yourself the question, "Could this be my heart?" and getting medical attention right away might save your life.

Risk Factors

The risk factors for heart disease are the same in men and women. But some of the patterns are different for women. Here's a brief overview:

- **High blood pressure.** At younger ages, men are more likely to have high blood pressure than women. But from the age of 65 onward, women are more likely to have high blood pressure than men.

- **High cholesterol.** Research shows that women are less likely than men to be aware that they have high cholesterol. It's important for women to get screened and, if necessary, to adjust their diets or begin medication.

- **Lack of exercise.** Women are more likely to be missing out on regular exercise. This is probably because many women are multitasking, balancing professional and personal responsibilities.

To reduce your risk of a heart attack, it's essential to manage these risk factors. Here are some guidelines:

Blood pressure. For generally healthy people, blood pressure is "high" when it's 140/90 or above. The top number—your *systolic blood pressure*—measures the pressure in your arteries when the heart contracts and pushes blood through the arteries to your body. The bottom number—the *diastolic pressure*—measures the pressure in your arteries when your heart is resting between beats. Normal is below 120/80, although the top number should be at least 90.

Cholesterol. Recommendations for cholesterol vary, but in general, a woman should aim to keep her cholesterol numbers in the following range:[5]

- Total cholesterol: below 200 mg/dL

- LDL cholesterol ("bad" cholesterol that increases your risk of a heart attack):
  - Below 160 mg/dL if your heart disease risk is low
  - Below 130 mg/dL if your heart disease risk is intermediate
  - Below 100 mg/dL if your risk is high, including if you have diabetes or you've already been diagnosed with heart disease

- HDL cholesterol ("good" cholesterol that lowers your risk of a heart attack): 50 mg/dL or above

Triglycerides. Triglycerides are a form of fat, and they're involved in storing energy. Your body won't work properly without them, but a high level in your blood can be a sign that your risk of heart disease is elevated. Your level should be less than 150 mg/dL.

Diabetes. If you have diabetes, you'll want to keep an eye on a test called hemoglobin A1C, which tells you how well your blood sugar has been controlled over the past few months. Most patients with diabetes should aim for an A1C below 7 percent.

Get checked for high blood pressure, abnormal cholesterol levels, and high triglycerides, and ask if you should be screened for diabetes. There are medications to treat each of these, and you may need to take them.

If you have your numbers on hand, you can use an online calculator to get an idea of your overall risk of having a heart attack in the next 10 years. Look for the Heart Attack Risk Assessment tool at the National Heart, Lung, and Blood Institute Web site. You'll need to enter your age, sex, total cholesterol, HDL cholesterol, and blood pressure, and whether you smoke or you take blood pressure medicine. It takes only about 5 minutes to complete.

http://hp2010.nhlbihin.net/atpiii/calculator.asp

This calculator won't work if you have diabetes or if you already have cardiovascular disease. If that's the case, you already know you're at a pretty high risk and should be taking precautions. To get a closer look, try the online calculator called Diabetes PHD (Personal Health Decisions) maintained by the American Diabetes Association. People without diabetes can use it, too.

**http://www.diabetes.org/living-with-diabetes
/complications/diabetes-phd/**

Reducing Your Risk

In addition to getting regular screenings for all of the risk factors listed on the previous pages, there are things that you can do to reduce your risk of heart disease.

Exercise. If you're not already physically active, get moving! You can walk, run, roller-skate, dance—whatever makes your heart beat faster. As a general rule, try to get at least 30 minutes of exercise at least 5 days a week. It doesn't have to be a heart-pounding game of tennis or a sprint on the exercise bike. Anything that increases your heart rate and makes you breathe a little harder will do.

Eat wisely. I know. You've heard it so many different times. But here are a few simple tips to consider when eating for heart health:

- Include a variety of fresh fruits and vegetables in your diet.

- Eat whole grain foods instead of foods made with processed white flour.

- Eat fish at least twice a week, because oily fish contains omega-3 fatty acids that might reduce your risk of dying from coronary artery disease. If you don't like fish, try omega-3 supplements.

- Cut back on the amount of saturated animal fats in your diet, which can lead to plaque in the arteries and result in cardiovascular problems.

- Cut back on salt to reduce your risk of high blood pressure. You should be getting less than 1,500 milligrams of sodium a day. A simple way to do this is to stop adding salt to meals and avoid processed foods, canned goods, and frozen meals.

Quit smoking. Smoking is a huge risk factor for heart disease. Smoking increases bad cholesterol while decreasing good cholesterol, promotes insulin resistance, and causes our blood vessels to constrict. Smoking also promotes inflammation of your body tissues, which is the underlying cause of many diseases. In addition, smoking causes a 50 percent increase in progression of plaques in our blood vessels.

If you smoke, find a quitting partner, get a nicotine patch, call your state's hotline—do whatever it takes to quit. If you're willing to try support from a trained counselor, call 1-800-QUITNOW or go to www.smokefree.gov. They'll link you to a network of

Women's Health: What's Normal and Not Normal As We Age

Normal	Not Normal
Hot flashes that last a few minutes at a time	Feeling hot and feverish all the time
Irregular menstrual periods	Periods that are extremely heavy or never seem to stop
Vaginal dryness	Losing control of your bladder
Noticing that your breasts don't seem as firm as they used to be	Noticing a lump in your breast or that your breasts have started to look uneven
Feeling your heart speed up when you exercise	Feeling chest pain when you exercise
Breaking a bone if you're in a car crash or other major accident	Breaking a bone because you bumped into something

state-based centers that exist specifically to help people quit smoking.

Get advice on aspirin. For some people, a low-dose aspirin every day can reduce the chance of a heart attack, stroke, or other problem due to cardiovascular disease. The reason I say "get advice" is because daily aspirin also carries risks: It can cause internal bleeding. You don't want to start taking it until you've talked it over with your doctor.

BONE HEALTH

Osteoporosis is a hidden disease—until one day it isn't. Unless you're tested for osteoporosis, the only way you'll know you have it is when a bone breaks. It could be your wrist, your hip, a rib . . . And if too many bones in your spine start to crumble, your posture will suffer. Permanently.

Case Study

Maryann is 50 years old, and she's a very busy woman. She's the president of the PTA at her daughter's school; she's active in a group that's training for a marathon; and she has a very successful business selling used bicycles online. She came in to see me because she'd been having hot flashes. "You have to help me," she said. "It's turning my life upside down."

Maryann said that frequently when she was leading a meeting or in the middle of an important work call, she'd suddenly break out into a sweat. "Not only do I completely lose my train of thought, but I think I'm scaring the younger girls at the office. They'll think that menopause makes you lose your mind!" Maryann is on the go constantly at work and at home, and time is tight. When she has to wait for a hot flash to go away, she feels like everything is getting off track. Sometimes a hot flash wakes her up at night, and then she's tired all the next day.

I asked her some questions about her menstrual cycles and her general health, and determined that her hot flashes were

I covered some details about osteoporosis in Chapter 2, so I won't rehash that information here. (Turn back to page 39 if you want to see what normal bone looks like compared with bone in someone with osteoporosis.) But this is a good place to explain the connection with menopause and to offer some more advice.

Why Is Osteoporosis a Concern after Menopause?

Your bones are living tissue. You may never have thought of bone in that way, but it is. Older bone is constantly being reabsorbed and renewed. In childhood and young adulthood, bones grow stronger and denser. Later on in life, bone renewal eventually stops

indeed a symptom of menopause. I suggested that she might want to try hormone therapy.

"I don't know, Dr. Whyte," Maryann said. "I've heard it's kind of dangerous. If I don't have time for these hot flashes, I certainly don't have time for a heart attack!"

I explained the current thinking about hormone therapy and safety. We discussed the various risks and benefits, and I reassured her that I would prescribe the lowest dose possible and that she wouldn't need to take this medicine forever.

Maryann decided to give it a try, and after a few months, her hot flashes became much less frequent. "It's manageable now, Dr. Whyte," she said. She also confided that since she'd been taking the hormones, she'd been enjoying sex with her husband more.

We decided to keep her on the therapy for a while longer. Most women who use hormone therapy for hot flashes can stop within a year, so I suggested she give it a few more months.

keeping up with bone loss. Bones become thinner as older tissue isn't completely replaced. As you go through menopause, the drop in estrogen speeds up bone loss.

Your risk of osteoporosis depends on your family history, your ethnic background, and your lifestyle. Some of the things that raise your risk include:

- Being white or Asian
- Being thin
- Having a close relative with osteoporosis
- Starting menopause early
- Not getting enough calcium
- Taking steroid medications for a long time

Staying Strong

Calcium is a major ingredient in your bones. You get calcium from the foods you eat, but a lot of women don't get enough. The chart below shows the recommended daily amount of calcium for women of various ages.

If you're not eating enough calcium-rich foods, you can take a calcium supplement. Just be sure you're getting about 15 minutes of sun exposure daily to help your body make adequate vitamin D, too. Your body needs vitamin D to make use of the calcium. Some calcium supplements actually contain vitamin D. You can find a wide variety of calcium supplements at the drugstore, including some that contain calcium carbonate, calcium citrate, or calcium phosphate. All of these should be effective as long as you take them with food. If that's not convenient, calcium citrate is your best bet.

Another important way to ward off osteoporosis is to get plenty of weight-bearing exercise. Weight-bearing exercise includes running, walking, dancing, and aerobics—basically anything that keeps you on your feet and working against gravity. Weight lifting counts, too. Swimming and biking are great exercise, but they're not considered weight-bearing. You've got to move some type of weight—either your own weight or a dumbbell.

A few other lifestyle changes that can help promote bone health include cutting down on your sodium intake (high levels of salt may speed up the loss of calcium from your bones), quitting smoking, and cutting back on alcohol and caffeine consumption.

Age	Calcium (milligrams)	Vitamin D (international units)
31–50	1,000	600
51–70	1,200 (women) 1,000 (men)	600
> 70	1,200	800

FIVE TIPS FOR MENOPAUSE AND BEYOND

1 Ask about help for menopause symptoms. You might not have any major symptoms—but if you do, and they're getting in the way of your life, talk with your doctor about hormone therapy and other options.

2 Get your blood pressure and cholesterol checked—and get them under control. If you've been ignoring high blood pressure or risky cholesterol levels, this is a great time to get serious about your numbers.

3 Get screened for breast cancer. Find out your personal risk of breast cancer. If you haven't been having regular mammograms and breast exams at the doctor's office, get started now.

4 Memorize the symptoms of a heart attack. It's not just chest pain. You might not even *have* chest pain! Learn what to look for—and if you ever think you may be having a heart attack, don't wait to get help.

5 Watch your calcium and vitamin D intake. Give some thought to your diet and lifestyle. Are you getting enough calcium from the foods you eat? Are you getting too little sun exposure for your body to make adequate vitamin D? If so, take a supplement.

Are Your Bones Normal?

Starting around age 65, it's a good idea for women to get an annual screening for osteoporosis. Men should start to be screened at age 70.

The screening tests for osteoporosis include a whole-body scan called a dual-energy x-ray absorptiometry scan. We call it DXA, or "dexa," for short. There are other tests that just check your heel bone or your hand, but you'll get the most useful results from a DXA.

If you do have osteoporosis, you may need to take medication to help strengthen your bones. Your doctor may also suggest medication if you don't yet have osteoporosis but are at high risk of developing it.

Most osteoporosis drugs slow down bone loss so that the renewal process has a chance to catch up. There are also drugs that promote the formation of new bone, but questions about safety mean that they're mainly an option for short-term use in people at high risk of breaking a bone.

If you have osteoporosis, you'll also need to:

• Pay attention to your diet. Make sure you're getting enough calcium from dairy items and foods such as kale and almonds.

• Plan a program of exercise that supports your bones without putting you in danger of a fracture. Your doctor can help you decide what's safe.

• Take a look around your house and make sure you don't have loose rugs, uneven steps, or other things that could cause you to fall.

• Get your eyesight and hearing checked. You don't want to trip or bump into something just because you couldn't see it well or didn't hear it coming.

• Make sure your muscles and nerves are in good shape. Numbness or weakness can put you at risk of a fall.

• Review your medications with your doctor, in case you're taking something that could make you dizzy or drowsy and increase your risk of falling.

Chapter 12

MALE MENOPAUSE: DOES IT EXIST?

True or False

Testosterone replacement is a cure for erectile dysfunction.　_____

Aging causes a 50 percent decrease in testosterone levels.　_____

Healthy males can make sperm into their eighties.　_____

All men go through a midlife crisis by the time they are 50.　_____

(Answers at end of chapter)

Have you been moody lately? Or maybe you've lost interest in sex? Do you feel weak and tired a lot?

You might be thinking these questions are geared toward women, but if you are a male and experiencing these symptoms, you might be going through "male menopause."

In recent years, we've started to learn that many men experience some of the same types of symptoms women do as they reach their forties and fifties. In men, it may be due to low testosterone.

I realize that a lot of men and even some doctors don't like the term *male menopause*. I agree, as it doesn't describe the problem very well and probably discourages men from discussing their symptoms. After all, what male would want to talk about having "menopause"? That doesn't seem normal.

Even though "menopause" includes the word "men," it means permanent cessation of the menses. So no matter how catchy the phrase "male menopause" might be, if you're not a woman, you can't experience menopause. There's another reason why "male menopause" isn't a very useful term, and that's because it's misleading. The hormonal changes that are associated with menopause in women happen fairly quickly. Once the processes surrounding a woman's menopause are complete, she no longer menstruates and her hormone levels are significantly and permanently changed. In men, the decrease in testosterone happens much more gradually, over the course of decades. There usually isn't one particular period of time when a man can say, "I'm going through 'the change'"—or a time when he can say, "Okay, that was it, my testosterone has now decreased."

Many doctors use the term *andropause* to describe the decrease in testosterone in a more medically appropriate way. You'll also see age-associated decreases in testosterone described as *partial androgen deficiency in aging men (PADAM)* or *late-onset hypogonadism (LOH)*. For men who seem to have symptoms, you'll see terms including *androgen deficiency syndrome of the aging male* and *symptomatic androgen deficiency (SAD)*.

LOW TESTOSTERONE

After the age of 60, 20 percent of men have low testosterone. After the age of 70, that number jumps to about 30 percent. Once men are 80, they have a 50 percent chance of experiencing a testosterone deficiency.

But what does it mean to have low testosterone? You might

have heard that when your testosterone level drops, so does your sex drive, your vitality, your muscle strength, your *joie de vivre.*

It's normal for a man's testosterone level to decline as he ages. When you're 60 or 70 or 80, you just don't have as much testosterone as you did when you were 20 or 30. But this doesn't have to mean an end to life as you know it. It also doesn't mean that you should expect to go through the same things that your wife or female friends may have experienced when their estrogen levels dropped during menopause. You probably don't have to brace yourself for mood swings or hot flashes. But you will experience some changes.

Before I explain the effects of low testosterone, I want to tell you a little bit about how your body makes testosterone and what it does. Then we'll look more closely at the changes in testosterone that happen as you age, the signs and symptoms that can be associated with low testosterone, and what's normally expected as we age, and what you can do if you think you have a problem.

Testosterone Basics

Culturally speaking, testosterone is the hormone that represents masculinity. When men try to one-up each other by bragging about their accomplishments in sports or at work, we say, "That's the testosterone talking." When a man has to have the fastest car or the biggest TV, we blame that on testosterone, too.

The medical reality is a little different. When a male baby is developing in the womb, testosterone and hormones made from it are essential for his body to develop male genitalia. When a boy reaches puberty, it is androgens, including testosterone, that cause him to grow pubic hair and make his testicles and penis develop into their adult shape and size. Androgens are also what make a boy's voice change and his face start to look like a man's. In adult men, testosterone is important to keep the sexual organs working properly. Within the testes, it is essential for making sperm.

So it sort of makes sense to think that if you have lots of testosterone, you're somehow more "manly" than a guy with a lower level, right? Well, it turns out that, within a pretty wide range of normal, guys have all kinds of testosterone levels. There might be some connections between testosterone levels and certain behaviors, like thrill seeking in young men, but for the most part, as long as your development during puberty was normal and you're healthy today, your testosterone levels probably don't have much to do with how much of a man you are. Your high school and college buddies simply were wrong!

Testosterone does a lot of other things in the body, beyond the development and maintenance of male physical characteristics. Various studies have found connections between testosterone levels and bone strength, muscle mass, metabolism, risk of diabetes, and even general quality of life. Testosterone may even have an influence on brain function.

Most of the testosterone in a man's body comes from the testes, from specific cells called *Leydig cells*. (A much smaller amount comes from the adrenal glands, which lie just above the kidneys.) The Leydig cells are regulated by hormones made in the pituitary gland, which sits way up in your skull at the base of your brain. And the pituitary gland itself gets messages from a part of the brain called the *hypothalamus*. The hypothalamus puts out a substance called *gonadotropin-releasing hormone (GnRH)*. GnRH tells the pituitary gland to start releasing *luteinizing hormone (LH)*, which travels through your body and tells the testes to get going and make some testosterone. When there is plenty of testosterone, the pituitary and hypothalamus reduce their signals. There are lots of other hormones, proteins, and other substances helping to regulate testosterone production, but this basic explanation should be enough to help you understand the changes that occur with aging and the idea of "male menopause." You can follow the hypothalamic-pituitary-testicular axis in the diagram below.

Declining Testosterone

As a man gets older, it's normal for his testosterone levels to decline. Starting around age 40, most men will experience a decline of

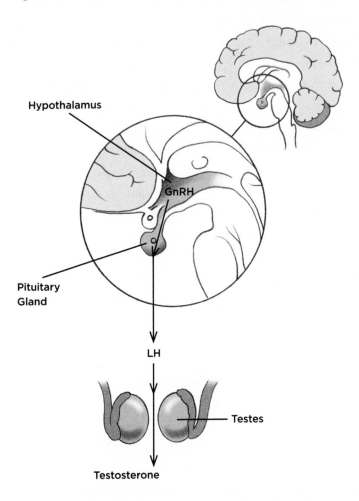

Hypothalamic-Pituitary-Testicular Axis—The hypothalamus receives signals from the brain to produce sperm and/or testosterone, causing it to signal the pituitary gland, which sends a unique signal to the testes and other glands involved in these processes.

about 1 percent per year in total testosterone. Just as with other conditions, individual men have their own unique patterns. Some might see their levels decline more quickly, others more slowly. Some men's levels never drop below what is considered "normal." Others become testosterone deficient, at least according to their laboratory reports, with no associated symptoms.

Medical researchers are trying to determine exactly why testosterone levels drop as men age. It could be a decline in testicular function, a change in the regulation by the pituitary gland and hypothalamus, or a combination of the two. Some recent research has tried to separate out the decline in testosterone due to aging from declines due to other medical problems that often occur as we get older, such as gaining excess weight. This research suggests that the age-related decline is more likely to be due to something changing in the testes, while an obesity-related decline is more likely due to a change in the body's regulation of testosterone. This sort of information might be useful in the future, because it could help us decide how to treat someone with signs or symptoms of low testosterone.

Many of my male patients have asked me if wearing tight underwear could have a negative impact on their testosterone levels. The answer is: absolutely not. Wearing tight underwear or pants may decrease sperm count, but sperm count and testosterone levels are two completely different issues. Your choice of underwear does not in any way impact your levels of testosterone.

Signs and Symptoms

Even as your testosterone levels decline over the years, you may not notice any adverse effects. And while there are symptoms associated with low testosterone, sometimes there can be other medical causes for these symptoms.

One symptom of low testosterone is *erectile dysfunction (ED)*. It's estimated that as many as 20 percent of men with ED have a testosterone deficiency. In these cases, ED medications such as Viagra and Levitra don't work effectively; so if you're taking one of these drugs and not seeing any results, it could be because you have low testosterone.

The following lists are adapted from guidelines created by the Endocrine Society, an organization dedicated to research on hormones and to the medical practice of endocrinology.[1] If you experience these symptoms, it's a good idea to go to your doctor and have your testosterone levels checked, as well as additional health screenings to rule out other possible causes.

- Reduced libido
- Decreased spontaneous erections
- Development of breast tissue
- Decreased body hair or the need to shave less often
- Small or shrinking testes
- Low sperm count (as measured by your doctor)
- A broken bone from mild injury, loss of height, or low bone density
- Hot flashes

The organization also suggests that your doctor consider checking your testosterone if you have some less specific signs and symptoms, too. Again, there are many possible causes for these signs and symptoms, so make sure to discuss them fully with your doctor.

- Decreased energy, loss of motivation, low initiative, or low self-confidence
- Depressed or "blue" mood

- Poor concentration or problems with memory
- Problems with sleep
- Anemia (low red blood cell count)
- A decrease in muscle strength or bulk
- An increase in body fat
- A decrease in performance at work or in physical tasks

Testing for Your Testosterone

If your doctor does think that your symptoms could be due to low testosterone, there are several different ways he or she may check your level. Bear in mind that many doctors aren't in agreement that low testosterone can be the cause of these symptoms, so you might need to speak up and ask for the test.

There are a few things you should know about the test. Much of the testosterone in your body is strongly bound to a protein called *sex hormone binding globulin (SHBG)*. About 2 percent is unbound, or "free," and about 60 percent is weakly bound to other proteins, including a common one called *albumin*. Together, the free and albumin-bound portions are known as *bioavailable testosterone*, meaning that the testosterone is available for the body to use.

One common test, "total testosterone," measures both the bound and free testosterone to give a single snapshot of the testosterone in your body. Sometimes, this test is all you need to make sure that your testosterone levels are within the range of normal. But it's important for you and your doctor to understand that it can also be misleading.

The problem is that a test for total testosterone doesn't really tell you how much testosterone is actually usable, or "free," within your body. If your total testosterone level is low-normal, and your level of SHBG is higher than usual, your free testosterone

might actually be low. Then again, with a low-normal total testosterone level and a normal or low level of SHBG, your body
might have access to all the testosterone it needs. Levels of SHBG
increase with age and also change with certain medical conditions, so if your total testosterone is on the low side, it may be
worth checking your free or bioavailable testosterone, too.

You should also talk with your doctor about the time of day the
test is performed. Testosterone levels change over the course of the
day, so experts often recommend checking testosterone in the morning to get the most consistent and appropriate measurement.

Other Reasons for Low Testosterone

Andropause is not the only reason a man's testosterone level might
be low. Low testosterone has also been associated with obesity and
other health problems, certain medications, and radiation and chemotherapy for cancer. It can also be caused by a tumor in the
pituitary gland. If you're having problems due to low testosterone,
don't just assume it's because you're getting older. Make sure to
talk with your doctor about all the possibilities.

Testosterone Supplementation

If you and your doctor decide that you could benefit from testosterone supplementation, you have several options. There are testosterone patches; there are gels you rub into your skin; there are
injections; and there is even a sort of pill that you tuck up against
your gums. Your doctor can help you decide which one is the best
choice for your medical needs and your lifestyle.

The safety of long-term testosterone supplementation isn't
known, and it's too complex a topic to cover in this book. So
just like with hormone replacement for women, we aim for the

Case Study

Fred is 67 years old. He was widowed in his forties and remarried at age 58. He says his wife is the best thing that ever happened to him—"And she's gorgeous, too!" Fred worked in construction most of his life until he retired 2 years ago. He has always been the upbeat one among his friends. He loves a good practical joke, and he and his friends like to play elaborate tricks on one another. When he retired, he knew he would have to make an effort to stay in shape, so he and his wife go to the gym together three times a week.

So when Fred came into my office complaining that he wasn't feeling right, I knew to pay attention. "I've been feeling out of sorts lately, doc," he said. "It's nothing really major, but I just don't have the energy I used to." He said he can still think up good practical jokes, but he doesn't have the oomph to put them together. At the gym, he felt frustrated. He was used to his workouts gradually getting easier over time, but lately, he just felt stuck. But the worst part, he confided, was that his marriage wasn't what it used to be. He seemed embarrassed to talk about it, but he finally admitted that he was talking about intimacy. "I'm not even sure if

smallest dose for the shortest period of time. When I treat patients for symptoms that could be due to low testosterone, I monitor their testosterone levels, red blood cell count, and prostate-specific antigen (PSA); turn to page 198 for PSA information.

There are also a few drawbacks and side effects to testosterone supplementation. It is not a good choice for men who plan to start or expand a family in the near future, as supplemental testosterone will actually make you less able to conceive a child. Also, if a patient has prostate cancer, I don't recommend supplemental testosterone, as it may worsen prostate cancer. Anytime I prescribe testosterone for a patient, I check in regularly to make sure that the treatment is actually working. If it doesn't alleviate my patient's symptoms, I stop the testosterone and look for other solutions.

the parts are still working," he said, because he just didn't feel much desire anymore. He couldn't say for sure when all this started. "Maybe in the last year or so?" he speculated.

There are a lot of things that could be going on with Fred. First, I screened him for depression and other illnesses. Maybe retirement wasn't agreeing with him. Anemia can cause low energy. All sorts of illnesses could be throwing him off his stride. As for the intimacy issues, I asked if anything had changed on an emotional level. Maybe he and his wife were having marital problems as they adjusted to their new lifestyle? I made sure I knew about any medicines he was taking. But I didn't discover anything that would cause his symptoms.

While I was ruling out the other possibilities, I went ahead and checked Fred's testosterone levels. It turns out that his free testosterone was low. I recommended a testosterone gel, and he agreed to give it a try. At his follow-up appointment, we rechecked his testosterone level, and it was back in the normal range. He said that the intimacy had returned to his marriage, and that he was feeling more energetic, both at the gym and in everyday life.

TESTOSTERONE AND PROSTATE CANCER

If a man develops prostate cancer, the treatment may include androgen deprivation therapy. Keeping levels of androgens, including testosterone, very low can slow the growth of a tumor or even cause it to shrink, at least for a while. Androgen deprivation therapy usually involves the use of drugs that shut down most of the body's production of testosterone; low testosterone levels can also be accomplished by surgically removing the testes. When it comes to testosterone supplementation, many people worry that giving a man extra testosterone could cause a tiny, as-yet-undetected tumor to start growing out of control. There has also been concern that testosterone supplementation could cause a new cancer to develop.

If your doctor diagnoses you with low testosterone and you want to try testosterone replacement therapy, how much should you worry about prostate cancer? No one knows for sure, but you need to be aware of the latest recommendations and you should ask questions. Some doctors believe that there isn't any risk, and that even men who have been treated for prostate cancer can use testosterone as long as the cancer seems to have been eradicated and the patients are carefully monitored. Other doctors hesitate to prescribe testosterone supplementation at all.

We're still waiting for a definitive answer. A few years ago, researchers examined 19 different studies of testosterone replacement therapy.[2] They looked at events such as prostate biopsies; elevated *prostate-specific antigen (PSA),* which can be a sign of prostate cancer; and prostate cancer diagnoses. (I'll explain more about PSA in the next section.) Taken all together, these events were more common in men who took testosterone. But when the researchers looked at prostate cancer by itself, the difference was small enough that, statistically speaking, it may have been just a coincidence.

One argument for safety is that testosterone supplementation isn't meant to raise your levels above what would be considered "normal," so it shouldn't be any riskier than having a normal testosterone level in the first place. A number of studies have looked for a connection between natural testosterone levels and prostate cancer, and the results have been mixed. They must have concluded that the data didn't show any link between testosterone levels and prostate cancer risk. However, research is ongoing. A very recent study suggests that there could be a connection between higher natural levels of free testosterone and more aggressive forms of prostate cancer, at least in men over age 65.[3] It remains to be seen what future studies will tell us.

The Endocrine Society's guidelines advise against giving testosterone replacement therapy to men with certain abnormalities of the prostate, such as nodules (bumps) that can be felt on a physical exam. A lump or bump on the prostate could be an undiagnosed cancer. An elevated PSA level would be a reason to hold off on prescribing testosterone, too.

Before trying testosterone supplementation, ask your doctor about the possible risks and side effects, and follow your doctor's instructions regarding follow-up tests and checkups.

SCREENING FOR PROSTATE CANCER

I said I'd explain more about PSA, and since we're on the topic of prostate cancer, this seems like a good place to do it. Prostate-specific antigen is a protein that's produced by the prostate gland, and it can be measured with a blood test. Certain prostate problems, including infection and an enlarged prostate, can cause your PSA level to rise. So can prostate cancer.

THREE TIPS TO INCREASE TESTOSTERONE NATURALLY

1 Hit the heavy weights. Numerous studies have shown that lifting heavy weights can increase testosterone levels for several days after an intense workout.

2 Consider eating foods rich in vitamin A, vitamin E, zinc, and carnitine. These vitamins and minerals have been shown to increase testosterone levels. Good sources include chicken, fish, avocados, pumpkin seeds, peanuts, almonds, and sweet potatoes.

3 Limit alcohol consumption to no more than two beers or glasses of wine daily. Drinking large amounts of alcohol does not make you manlier; in fact, it will decrease testosterone levels.

For many years, PSA testing has been used as a screening method to check for prostate cancer. Many doctors do this test routinely as part of an annual physical. We all know that catching cancer early can be lifesaving, so this sounds like a great idea, right?

Actually, it's a lot more complicated. Prostate cancer is pretty common, and in fact the American Cancer Society estimates that a man's lifetime risk of being diagnosed with prostate cancer is about one in six.[4] This cancer can be a killer. About 30,000 men die of it each year, and more than 90 percent of these men are middle-aged and older. But prostate cancer can also grow very, very slowly. Autopsy studies have shown that it is not uncommon for men to have prostate cancer and never even know it or be affected by it. We are starting to figure out which prostate cancers are likely to be dangerous and which ones are likely to be less harmful.

If the treatment for prostate cancer were more straightforward, then it would make sense to screen every man and automatically treat every cancer that was diagnosed. In fact, the treatments that are usually recommended have important side effects, including a risk of causing impotence. Depending on the treatment, other potential complications include urinary incontinence and bowel problems. If the cancer appears to carry a very low risk of spreading, one option is to hold off on treatment and just keep an eye on things, with regular tests to be sure the cancer isn't growing. We used to call this watchful waiting, but that sounded too much like we weren't doing anything, so now we call it active surveillance. For a lot of men, though, "low risk" prostate cancer is just as scary as any other cancer. They want it out of their bodies, no matter what. And that means some men are undergoing surgery, chemotherapy, or radiation treatment when, if they hadn't had a screening test, they likely would have been just fine.

Another concern about using PSA testing to screen for prostate cancer is the fact that cancer isn't the only thing that causes elevated levels. Many men will end up with a lot of worry, not to mention the discomfort of a prostate biopsy, only to find out that they're just fine. Then again, when a PSA test catches a dangerous, high-risk cancer, screening seems like a very good idea indeed.

Because of this balance between the potential for saving lives and the risk of unnecessary biopsies and treatments, many expert organizations now recommend that men talk it over with their doctors before undergoing a PSA test. Once you have a better understanding of the potential risks and benefits, you can make the decision that's right for you.

The American Cancer Society has some recommendations for screening that I think make a lot of sense. The following advice is based on their screening guidelines:[5]

- First, talk with your doctor. Make sure you understand what screening can and can't accomplish and what will happen if your test is positive.

- Most men should have this discussion starting at age 50. Men at high risk should start earlier, at age 45; this includes African Americans and men whose fathers or brothers had prostate cancer before age 65. If you have a strong family history of prostate cancer, such as several close relatives who were diagnosed before age 65, start at age 40.

- If you choose screening, it should involve a PSA test and may also include a *digital rectal exam (DRE)*. For a DRE, your doctor will insert a gloved finger into your rectum and feel the surface of your prostate to check for any lumps or other abnormalities.

- The schedule for future screening tests will depend on your PSA level.

- Over the years, continue to talk with your doctor about the pros and cons of prostate cancer screening. It's likely that new information will become available, and you'll want to know if anything important has changed.

FOUNTAIN OF YOUTH?

If it's true that testosterone can make men feel stronger, livelier, and sexier—and even help with erectile dysfunction—wouldn't it make sense to give all older men the option of supplementing their decreasing testosterone?

It might, if we knew for sure that it would make a difference, and that there weren't better, safer ways to achieve the same results. But we just don't have that evidence yet. We also don't know what risks might be involved in giving testosterone to otherwise healthy men. For now, though, I don't know about you, but I'd prefer to avoid testosterone supplements if I'm not 100 percent sure I need them.

Male Menopause: What's Normal and Not Normal As We Age	
Normal	**Not Normal**
Having a little extra fat on your body, relative to muscle	Developing breast tissue
Sympathizing with a female spouse or partner who's having hot flashes	Having hot flashes yourself
Losing some strength or muscle bulk if you haven't been exercising lately	Losing strength or muscle bulk without a good reason
Recognizing that you don't have the energy you did when you were 21	Feeling like you don't have any energy at all

Answers to true/false statements: False, True, True, False

MENTAL HEALTH

You might be surprised to learn that the prevalence of most mental health problems actually decreases as we get older. The elderly have *lower* rates of mental health problems compared with the middle-aged. Why is this?

Some researchers have suggested that constant exposure to adverse experiences gradually creates resistance to the psychological effects of such experiences—a so-called *psychological immunization*.[1] Let me put this in "nondoctor talk": When you endure many difficult life experiences (e.g., loss of a job, death of a family member, trauma), you actually build up resiliency. It's similar to being vaccinated against a disease—a little pain now, but you're able to handle a more serious problem later on.

However, mental health problems can and do develop as we get older. Nearly 20 percent of people 55 years of age and older experience mental disorders that are not part of normal aging. It's important to recognize what is normal and what is not normal since there are effective treatments for mental health problems. The most common psychological problems that can occur as we approach middle age include depression, anxiety, and cognitive impairment (any decrease in mental function).

Dementia is another mental health disorder that can develop in our older years; turn to page 83 for more information on dementia.

SPECTRUM OF MENTAL HEALTH

Do you remember when characters with mental illness were portrayed in television and film as either the perpetrators of violence or the victims of violence? They were hidden away in state asylums or made into dangerous villains and psycho killers. We've come a long way in recent years in how we regard mental illness in our culture. Now, characters with mental illness are often portrayed as likeable and active members of society.

These changes in thinking about mental illness are likely due to the evolving understanding of mental illness. The stigma of mental illness is not gone, but it has been reduced. At the same time, mental illness is much more common than one might imagine. The National Institute of Mental Health reports that every year, one in four adults, nearly 60 million Americans, experiences a mental health disorder. Most of us know someone with mental illness or might have experienced a bout of mental illness ourselves. The reality is that mental illness represents a spectrum where most people function well in society.

I remember when patients would be embarrassed to bring up issues of depression, post-traumatic stress disorder, obsessive-compulsive disorder, or any other mental health topic. Now, as part of medical training, physicians are taught to actively inquire about our patients' mental health. And many clinics and hospitals have instituted mental health screens to make sure we catch any problems early on. Unfortunately, getting rid of stigma does not cure mental illness. Much work remains to be done in the areas of research, diagnosis, treatment, and prevention.

DO YOU FEEL SAD ALL THE TIME?

You noticed the change right away. Within a month of your mother's 80th birthday, she lost interest in her appearance, gave up on reading the newspapers, and started staying in bed half the day instead of getting up for her usual 6:00 a.m. coffee. Always vivacious, she became increasingly withdrawn. Your sister said it was just a normal part of aging, but you didn't accept that. You called her doctor, who diagnosed depression and prescribed a low dose of an antidepressant. Within 6 weeks, she was almost back to her usual self.

Good for you! You weren't taken in by the "normal part of aging" line. Data show that depression is not inevitable in the elderly.

I need to point out that sadness and grief are normal responses to life events that occur with aging, such as the loss or change of a job, death of a spouse or other loved one, change in housing situation, change in financial situation, or simply numerous physical ailments. However, such sadness or grief should not last all day, every day for several months or more.

Untreated depression can be particularly dangerous in the elderly. Did you know that the highest suicide rate in the United

States is among men who are 85 or older? Depression often makes it hard for people to take proper care of themselves, as well, which can worsen underlying health conditions.

When any of my patients say that an elderly parent sleeps all day, stops doing things they've always enjoyed, avoids spending time with the grandchildren or great-grandchildren, isn't picking up after him or herself anymore, isn't eating well, or is pulling away from them, I always suspect depression. Depression is one of the most easily treated forms of mental illness, so don't let yourself or your loved ones lose time that could be spent enjoying the pleasures of life.

There are some risk factors for depression that you should be aware of. These include:

- Poorly managed pain
- Difficulty sleeping
- Social isolation
- Widowed, divorced, or separated
- Lower socioeconomic status
- Multiple medical conditions
- Functional impairment

Sometimes it seems that risk factors can be a little like "the chicken or the egg." After all, if you have trouble sleeping, you could become depressed; or being depressed could cause difficulty in sleeping. The important point is to realize they are related. Depression can be rather difficult to spot as we get older. As we age, our health needs become more complicated. Medical problems such as high blood pressure, heart disease, osteoporosis, and arthritis are common and can mask the emotional challenges that we or our loved ones face, until they have reached a critical stage.

Mental Health: What's Normal and Not Normal As We Age	
Normal	**Not Normal**
Couple days of sadness	Long-term depression
Anxiety about an upcoming special event	Obsessive-compulsive thoughts
More time needed to learn new materials	Trouble concentrating
Desire to be organized	Consumed by need for routine

GERIATRIC DEPRESSION SCALE

There is a very good questionnaire that doctors often use to diagnose depression in people over the age of 60. It consists of five questions:

1. Are you basically satisfied with your life?
2. Do you often get bored?
3. Do you often feel helpless?
4. Do you prefer staying at home rather than going out and doing new things?
5. Do you feel pretty worthless the way you are now?

Two out of five depressive responses ("no" to question 1 and/or "yes" to questions 2 through 5) suggest the diagnosis of depression.

Many middle-aged and elderly patients will benefit from numerous effective therapies for depression, such as medications as well as psychotherapy, sometimes referred to as "talk therapy." Both of these therapeutic interventions have been proven to be successful in the young as well as the very old. There may need to be some adjustments in dosages as we get older, but treatment can still be very effective.

FIVE TIPS FOR MENTAL HEALTH

1 Make sure you and your loved ones develop hobbies. Hobbies are a way to allow your mind to decompress and not always be focused on work and personal issues.

2 Stay connected. Maintaining relationships has been shown to reduce mental health problems. It's not the quantity of the connections, but rather the quality of the connections that matters.

3 Don't be too proud to seek and accept support for yourself and others. Talk with your doctor about mental health problems.

4 Accept change. The French have a saying, *Plus ça change, plus c'est la même chose*—the more things change, the more they stay the same. The fact is that life changes—a lot—especially as we move through the decades. Be open to change.

5 Reduce stress. I know you cannot eliminate stress, but there are ways to reduce it, and you often have to consciously and actively find these ways. Many have already been discussed in earlier chapters; they include eating healthy, being active, forging relationships, and taking vacations.

TROUBLE PAYING ATTENTION?

When it comes to Attention Deficit Hyperactivity Disorder (ADHD), people tend to fall into one of two camps: One camp seems to think it's a completely made-up disorder, while the other camp thinks practically everyone has some form of it. As a physician, I do know this disorder exists; at the same time, though, I do think the term has been overused.

So what exactly is ADHD?

ADHD is an illness characterized by inattention, hyperactivity, and impulsivity. There are three different types of the disorder: inattentive, hyperactive/impulsive, and combined.

Although ADHD is usually diagnosed in childhood, it is not a disorder limited to children—ADHD often persists into adulthood and is frequently not diagnosed until later years. If you were diagnosed with childhood ADHD, chances are you have carried at least some of the symptoms into adulthood. However, it is unusual to be newly diagnosed with ADHD past 40 years of age.

To meet the formal diagnostic criteria of ADHD, an individual must display: (1) at least six inattentive-type symptoms for the inattentive type; (2) at least six hyperactive-type symptoms for the hyperactive/impulsive type; (3) all of the above to have the combined type.

I've listed the symptoms for each type of ADHD in the chart below. Each of these symptoms, when experienced alone, is fairly common. But when combined, they can be problematic.

Older patients often ask me if they might have ADHD because they have been having trouble concentrating. It's not uncommon to have some trouble concentrating as you get older, but that

Inattentive Type	Hyperactive/Impulsive Type
Indecisive	Easily bored without constant activity
Poor organization skills	
Trouble beginning tasks on time	Avoids sedentary work
	Seeks stimulating work
Trouble completing tasks on time	Often chooses to work multiple jobs or long hours
Inability to shift tasks	Impatient
Avoiding activities that require continued concentration	Impulsive
	Quickly loses temper
Procrastination	Easily frustrated
Inability to handle multiple activities at once	
Unreliable	

Source: Katragadda, S., and H. Schubiner. ADHD in children, adolescents, and adults. *Primary Care: Clinics in Office Practice* 34 (2007): 317–41.

doesn't mean you have ADHD. The speed of our brain synapses slows down slightly as we age. I've experienced this recently while trying to learn a foreign language; I can tell you it's been harder than I thought. If you or an elderly parent is having trouble concentrating, don't jump to conclusions.

DID I LOCK THE CAR?

Perhaps you have to check a few times to make sure you locked your car door. Or your father has to line up all his books from tallest to shortest on his bookshelf. Most of the time, this kind of nitpicky behavior is perfectly normal. One should start to worry when such behaviors become so consuming that they interfere with daily life.

Obsessive-Compulsive Disorder (OCD) certainly has become more well known in recent years; it's even become part of society's parlance. But the truth is that OCD is not common; only about 2 percent of the population suffers from it at some point in time. And as we approach middle age, the incidence of new diagnoses becomes even less common.

How do you know if you or a loved one has OCD? Typically, look for three things:

1. The person has obsessions.
2. He or she does compulsive behaviors.
3. The obsessions and compulsions take a lot of time and get in the way of important activities the person values, such as going to work, going to school, spending time with family and friends, and participating in hobbies.

Obsessions are involuntary, seemingly uncontrollable thoughts, images, or impulses that occur over and over again in your mind.

The problem is that you don't want to have these ideas—in fact, you know that they don't make any sense. But you can't stop them.

Compulsions are behaviors or rituals that you feel driven to act out again and again. Usually, compulsions are performed in an attempt to make obsessions go away. For example, if you're obsessed with germs, you may wash your hands hundreds of times throughout the day. However, the relief never lasts. In fact, the obsessive thoughts might come back stronger after a compulsive act. And the compulsive behaviors often end up causing anxiety as they become more demanding and time-consuming—making it difficult to hold a job or maintain a relationship.

When people have OCD, they recognize that their obsessive thoughts and compulsive behaviors are unreasonable and irrational, but even so, they feel unable to resist them and break free.

When I'm considering the possibility of OCD in a patient, I typically ask two questions:

1. Are there certain thoughts that go through your mind over and over that you cannot get rid of?
2. Are there habits or actions that you feel compelled to repeat?

If the patient answers "yes" to both questions, he or she may have OCD and need further testing.

Symptoms typically begin during childhood or the early twenties. Like ADHD, it would be very unusual to first start developing symptoms when someone is in their fifties, sixties, or seventies. That doesn't mean that it cannot happen, but other reasons for behavior changes in adults and the elderly should be considered. However, if someone has already been diagnosed with OCD in young adulthood, it can get worse as one becomes older. They likely will need adjustments of their medications.

Case Study

Charlie is a 55-year-old patient who comes in about every 2 years for follow-up appointments. He doesn't come in annually because, as he says, "I don't want to bother you, Doctor Whyte. There are a lot more sick people than me out there." He's in pretty good health, with the exception of high blood pressure and elevated triglycerides. He takes a beta-blocker for his blood pressure and uses an omega-3 supplement for his triglycerides.

At a recent visit, he complained about occasional headaches. He noted they occur a few times a week, typically in the front of his head; they don't go anywhere and they last for about 30 minutes. They often go away with aspirin or simply rest. Charlie doesn't have any history of migraines and doesn't have any other complaints. He does tell me that he recently was laid off from his job, but "I've been wanting to quit for a while, so I was happy getting a severance."

Charlie's headaches didn't seem to be too severe and didn't raise any red flags for me. So I asked him to keep a headache log, and I recommended that he take naproxen for the pain. I also asked him to come back in 2 weeks.

At the next visit, he said his headaches hadn't changed and, in fact, seemed to be occurring a little more often. Charlie had

DOESN'T EVERYONE GET ANXIOUS?

It's normal to be anxious at certain times in your life, especially around big events and important occasions. However, many people suffer from anxiety that occurs nearly every day; that is not normal, even if you have a lot of stress in your life.

Generalized anxiety disorder (GAD) is characterized by excessive worry and anxiety that is difficult to control and causes significant distress and impairment. The actual medical definition says "excessive anxiety and worry about a number of events or

been unemployed almost 4 months. I asked him if he'd been feeling depressed, and he said, "Doc, I never get depressed." So I asked him the questions from the depression questionnaire on page 207. He answered "yes" to most of the questions, but then said, "Doesn't everyone feel that way sometimes? Besides, I have no job and it's a tough economy out there. Who wouldn't get a little depressed?"

I pointed out that it's okay to get depressed and that he has had a tough year in terms of job loss. But I also emphasized that it's not normal to have depression for this extended period of time, even if he is unemployed. I suggested that his headaches may actually be related to depression. Charlie wasn't convinced, so I adjusted his naproxen dose and asked him to come back in a week. "If I'm still having headaches then, I'll try a depression pill," Charlie said.

At his next appointment, he said he was still having the headaches. I started him on a low dose of an antidepressant, and I also switched his beta-blocker, which can cause depression, to lisinopril. He came back again in 4 weeks, with little improvement. I increased the dose of his antidepressant, and within 2 months, he said he was feeling much better, and his headaches had gone away.

activities, occurring more days than not for at least 6 months, that are out of proportion to the likelihood or impact of feared events." That seems like it could be somewhat subjective, so I often use a seven-item anxiety questionnaire.

A score of 5 – 9 = mild anxiety; 10 – 14 = moderate anxiety; 15 – 21 = severe anxiety.

Twice as many women as men suffer from anxiety. It's important to recognize generalized anxiety disorder because there are effective treatments. Sometimes women think anxiety is just part of their gender or part of the aging process; it's neither.

Generalized Anxiety Disorder (GAD) 7

Over the last 2 weeks, how often have you been bothered by the following problems?

Problems	Not at all	Several days	More than half the days	Nearly every day
1. Feeling nervous, anxious, or on edge	0	1	2	3
2. Not being able to stop or control worrying	0	1	2	3
3. Worrying too much about different things	0	1	2	3
4. Trouble relaxing	0	1	2	3
5. Being so restless that it is hard to sit still	0	1	2	3
6. Becoming easily annoyed or irritable	0	1	2	3
7. Feeling afraid, as if something awful might happen	0	1	2	3
*Total Score _____ =	Add columns.	_____ +	_____ +	_____

If you checked off any problems, how difficult have these problems made it for you to do your work, take care of things at home, or get along with other people?

Circle one:	Not difficult at all	Somewhat difficult	Very difficult	Extremely difficult

*Refer to bottom of page 213 to decipher your score.

Source: *Spitzer, RL, Kroenke, K, Williams, JB, Lowe, B. A brief measure for assessing generalized anxiety disorder: the GAD-7. Arch Intern Med 2006; 166:1092*

PHYSICAL SYMPTOMS AND DRUGS

Remember that mental health issues can present as physical symptoms. Physicians often spend a great deal of time and resources working-up physical symptoms and don't take time to screen for mental health. So be sure to consider depression and anxiety when new physical problems arise.

Drugs—including prescription, over-the-counter, illicit, and supplements—all have the potential to cause mental health problems. As we get older, our bodies often don't eliminate some drugs as quickly as they should, or we simply respond differently than we did when we were younger. If you suddenly start to feel a little "off" or notice that an elderly parent or spouse is behaving strangely, consider any new medications that have recently been started and talk with a doctor.

Chapter 14

DRUGS AND ALCOHOL

True or False

People over the age of 60 are less likely to
become addicted to drugs or alcohol.   _____

Pain relievers are the most commonly abused
prescription drug.   _____

It's recommended to drink a glass of red wine daily
since it may reduce your chance of a heart attack.   _____

Narcotics should be the last choice for pain relief.   _____

(Answers at end of chapter)

I have a question for you: Can an older person become an addict? We often associate drug abuse or alcoholism with the lifestyle of young people, but as we age, the tendency to misuse all kinds of drugs, including prescription pain relievers and alcohol, can actually increase. After all, as we approach middle age and beyond, we are likely to be using some prescription medications. The same is true for alcoholism, which can worsen with age, and can be a frequent cause of death among seniors.

So how do you know when you or a loved one has a problem? And if you've always enjoyed having a glass or two of wine at dinner or a couple of beers in the evening to relax, how can you tell if you are still able to "hold your liquor" or if it's time to cut back? Do your medication dosages need to be adjusted once you pass age 50?

WHAT COUNTS AS ABUSE

I'm sure you've heard the line "the person who drinks more than me is the one who has the problem." Most people who abuse drugs or alcohol do not think they have a problem. We do, though, have a standard definition of what constitutes abuse.

Abuse is defined as using the medication or substance (e.g., alcohol) in a manner that deviates from medical, legal, and social standards.

Nearly 8 million people use prescription drugs for purposes other than those prescribed. That's actually more people than those who use such illegal drugs as cocaine, heroin, and methamphetamines combined. Prescription medications are second only to marijuana as an abused substance. As people age, there is a decline in the use of illegal drugs but an increase in the abuse of prescription drugs. Nearly one in five seniors abuses prescription drugs or alcohol. The most commonly abused prescription drugs are opiates, sedatives, and painkillers. No one is abusing their cholesterol or blood pressure medications!

The high incidence of prescription drug abuse can make it challenging for me as a doctor to help my aging patients with pain relief. While I'm concerned about preserving their quality of life, I'm also concerned about the hazards of addiction as well as accidental overdose. As we age, our bodies do not eliminate medications as quickly or as easily, and they stay present in our bloodstreams longer. By the time we're 70, dosages usually need to be adjusted—sometimes even cut in half. As we age, we are also often taking many different medications that have the potential to interact with each other and cause problems. I know that many of my colleagues are undertreating anxiety disorders, sleeping problems, and chronic pain in their patients because they're reluctant to prescribe medications with abuse potential. It's a balance of competing goals—maximizing therapy while at the same time minimizing risk of dependence.

It certainly is normal to take multiple medications as we get older, especially antidepressants and pain relievers. And as I discussed in previous chapters, medications are often effective and necessary as we age. But it's not normal to be dependent upon them.

What do I mean by "dependent"? Here are some criteria to define dependence:

- Recurrent substance use in physically hazardous situations (e.g., while driving)
- Recurrent legal problems related to drug or alcohol use
- Failure to fulfill work or social obligations
- Continued use despite drug- or alcohol-related social or interpersonal problems

It is quite challenging to wean yourself from a medication once you become dependent, and it should not be attempted without medical supervision. As we get older, we do not always understand how drugs will impact our bodies or might not recognize the impact they are having on our bodies. For instance, our bodies can become dependent on antianxiety medications such as Valium or Xanax. We may not even realize it until we try to stop the medication. Other medications may actually lower our blood pressure without us even being aware of it; when we stop the medication, our blood pressure can increase to levels that are dangerously high.

It can be difficult to recognize signs of prescription drug dependence, as they are often similar to the signs of normal aging. Mood swings, memory loss, loss of interests, difficulty sleeping, change in weight, excess sweating, and shaking or tremors are all typical symptoms of substance abuse. These symptoms usually

Substance Use: What's Normal and Not Normal As We Age	
Normal	**Not Normal**
One glass of wine most days of the week	Two or three glasses of wine every day
Multiple prescription drugs for chronic medical conditions	Legal troubles involving narcotics
Medication for pain relief managed by a doctor	Borrowing medication or lying about refills

develop over a short period of time—weeks or months—versus symptoms associated with normal aging, which occur gradually, over years. Drug dependence in the elderly is especially dangerous because it often leads to falls and accidental overdoses.

ALCOHOL—IT'S DIFFERENT AS WE GET OLDER

It's normal to enjoy wine and alcohol. And there are data that show moderate consumption is probably healthy for the heart. As we get older, our consumption of alcohol is certainly different than it was when we were younger.

It is not normal to drink excessively as you approach middle age. Perhaps once a year you get a little too merry at the annual neighborhood Christmas party, but getting drunk on a frequent basis simply is not normal. I'm sure you have also noticed that it takes less alcohol to make you feel tipsy as you get older. As we age, our bodies don't rid themselves of alcohol as quickly or as easily. The toxins stay in our bloodstreams longer, and we become intoxicated more quickly and with fewer drinks. By the time you reach 60, the amount of alcohol that it takes to make you feel drunk can decrease by a third.

THREE TIPS TO PREVENT SUBSTANCE ABUSE

1 Choose your "surroundings" carefully. If you surround yourself with people who drink a lot of alcohol or abuse prescription drugs, you are more likely to engage in that behavior as well. The role of family is also critical in prevention.

2 Ask your physician questions about any potentially addictive drugs you have been prescribed. Especially if you've struggled with addictions in the past, talk with your doctor about the size of your dosage and the duration of time you need to take it. You do want your medical conditions treated effectively, but you also do not want your body to become dependent.

3 Dispose of drugs—especially narcotics—that you or your loved one used for a short time. Many people will use sleeping pills or narcotics if they happen to still be in the house. If they're not around, you cannot use them, or you'll need to call the doctor and explain why you need a refill.

Alcohol is one of those areas where too much of a good thing can be harmful as we get older. As I mentioned earlier, moderate alcohol consumption does offer some health benefits, but at some point it does more harm than good.

THE FRENCH PARADOX

Have you heard of the French paradox? It refers to the fact that the rate of heart disease in France is lower than we would expect given the French lifestyle, which typically includes eating rich foods and drinking wine daily.

Some researchers attribute the low incidence of heart disease to red wine consumption. Red wine contains phenols and flavonoids, which we believe have antioxidant properties. Red wine also contains resveratrol, which is a substance produced by plants; it is found in the skin of grapes. Some studies show that it may prevent blood clots; others have shown that it seems to extend the life of mice. That is always very encouraging, but remember, we're not mice! Some patients have asked me if they should take resveratrol supplements. I don't recommend it; we just do not have enough data yet.

Does the French paradox mean you should drink red wine at dinner every night? Probably not. The French, as well as many other Europeans, have a totally different style of living that likely contributes to lower heart disease. It's not just the consumption of wine.

ALCOHOL ABUSE

Approximately 10 percent of the population abuses alcohol. This includes many people in middle age and older. Some people believe that alcohol abuse only starts in the twenties and thirties. That's a myth. A large percentage of adults first develop drinking problems in their forties, fifties, and sixties.

Problem drinking reduces the quality of life for patients and their families. How do you know when drinking has become a problem?

Here are a couple of questionnaires that physicians often use, that you can use as well:

AUDIT-C

1. How often did you have a drink containing alcohol in the past year?

Never	0 point
Monthly or less	1 point
2–4 times a month	2 points
2–3 times per week	3 points
4 or more times a week	4 points

Case Study

Jason is a 71-year-old widower. He has multiple health problems, including congestive heart failure and severe arthritis. Due to his limited ability to get around, he lives with his daughter, Clare, who functions as a caregiver. Last winter, Jason slipped outside on the ice and broke his right wrist. He underwent surgical repair but had a difficult time at rehabilitation. He was on a small dose of daily morphine to help with pain, since he said Motrin, naproxen, and even Vicodin upset his stomach.

When he came in to see me, he said his pain was worsening. I decided to increase the dose of his morphine, and I ordered additional physical therapy. Jason called me a couple of days after the appointment to tell me that he'd dropped the prescription bottle in the sink and the pills fell down the drain. I'm usually a bit suspicious of stories like this, but I've known Jason a long time and believed him to be honest.

Two months after that, Jason returned for a follow-up appointment with Clare. He seemed a bit disheveled, and Clare said he'd

2. How many drinks did you have on a typical day when you were drinking in the past year?

1 or 2	0 point
3 or 4	1 point
5 or 6	2 points
7 to 9	3 points
10 or more	4 points

3. How often did you have five or more drinks on occasion in the past year?

Never	0 point
Less than monthly	1 point
Monthly	2 points
Weekly	3 points
Daily or almost daily	4 points

been having trouble sleeping. "Could you give him a sleeping pill?" she asked. I suspected the lack of sleep might be related to his pain, so I asked how he's been managing his pain. "That's another thing," Clare remarked. "I don't think the pain meds are strong enough." Over the next 6 months, Jason came in several more times with additional health complaints. I grew concerned because he had been on pain medication for a relatively long period of time after wrist surgery. After talking with Jason and Clare in more detail and screening Jason for drug dependence, it became clear to me that he'd become dependent on the morphine.

Although he still had some pain, I slowly tapered him off of the morphine dosage while at the same time adding a nonsteroidal anti-inflammatory medication as well as Tylenol for pain relief. I also had him resume physical therapy three times a week. Within 6 weeks, he was off all narcotics and doing much better, with very little pain.

In men, a total score of 4 or more is considered positive and the person needs help. In women, a total score of 3 or more is considered positive.

Sometimes I even shorten the questionnaire to:

How many times in the past year have you consumed x or more drinks in a day?

x = 5 for men and x = 4 for women

If the answer is more than once, I then ask more questions. You may have heard of the CAGE questionnaire.[1] This is also a set of questions (shown on the following page) that you can ask to help determine if there is potential abuse.

1. Have you ever felt the need to cut down on drinking?

2. Have you ever felt annoyed by criticisms of your drinking?

3. Have you ever had guilty feelings about your drinking?

4. Do you ever take a morning eye opener (a drink first thing in the morning to steady your nerves or get rid of a hangover)?

One "yes" response suggests the need for closer examination.

HOW MUCH IS TOO MUCH?

Moderate alcohol consumption is considered "normal," but how do you know what's considered moderate and what's excessive? The guidelines below suggest healthy limits for alcohol consumption:

- For healthy men up to age 65: no more than 4 drinks in a day and no more than 14 drinks in a week
- For healthy men over age 65: no more than 3 drinks in a day and no more than 7 drinks in a week
- For all women, independent of age: no more than 3 drinks in a day and no more than 7 drinks in a week

Those are the maximum amounts. By no means are those the amounts you should strive for. After the age of 65, especially, men and women should be cautious about alcohol consumption; a normal limit is about 1 or 2 drinks a day.

There are effective treatments for alcohol abuse. The key is to recognize the abuse and develop a comprehensive treatment strategy.

Answers to true/false Statements: False, True, True, False

A TRIP to THE HOSPITAL

Each year, nearly one of five adults will visit the emergency room. Care in a hospital can save your life—or at least reduce pain and prevent more serious health problems. The decision to go to the hospital is not an easy one, and as we get older, we're often even more reluctant to go. I'm sure you have struggled just as I have with aging parents who refuse to go to the doctor or to the hospital when they are having a problem. Many people are fearful of hospitals, especially older folks who grew up in an age when people who went to hospitals often didn't leave. That's clearly not the case for hospitals anymore, but long-held perceptions can remain.

Issues of insurance, wait time, child care, elder care, transportation, and more also factor into the decision. But your health is your most important asset. If you feel you need to go to the hospital, then go. You can work out all the other issues later. Especially in your older years, it's important to err on the side of caution. I've seen too many bad outcomes from folks who said, "I'm sure it's nothing" when it actually turned out to be something serious.

But while a visit to the hospital can save your life, it can also be hazardous to your health. That's right, you read that sentence correctly: Hospitals can be dangerous places. Nearly 100,000 people die each year due to preventable errors made in the hospital. These include infections, problems with anesthesia, incorrect surgical procedures, and wrong medications.

So how do you maximize the benefits of being in the hospital while minimizing any harm? The best way to approach a stay in the hospital is to think of it in three phases: before the hospital visit, during the hospital visit, and after the hospital visit.

BEFORE THE HOSPITAL VISIT

If you're reading this book, you will have likely spent some time in a hospital either as a patient or as a caregiver for a loved one. If you haven't yet spent any significant time in a hospital, it's likely that you will in the next few years, so it's important to be prepared.

One of the most important things you can do to prepare yourself or a loved one for a stay in the hospital is to assemble your medical information, identification, and insurance information in one place. You might come to the hospital incapacitated, or you simply might be too stressed to think clearly. I have seen many people forget basic information such as their date of birth with all the commotion in a hospital. So have a piece of paper ready to hand to the doctors and nurses you meet.

What should be on the piece of paper? Of course, you should

list all of your prescription medications, including the dosages. Also list any supplements or vitamins as well as over-the-counter medications (e.g., Tylenol, aspirin, Tums) you might be taking. We tend to forget that these often can have harmful interactions with prescription medicines we are taking. For instance, my mother takes Coumadin, a blood thinner. All sorts of medications, supplements, and vitamins can affect how well Coumadin thins her blood. Also list any allergies you have to medications or anesthesia. Include your medical conditions (e.g., high blood pressure, diabetes, heart attacks) and any recent surgeries (e.g., knee replacement, gallbladder surgery, stent placement in blood vessels). Below is a list of essential information you shouldn't forget when taking a trip to the hospital:

- Name
- Date of Birth
- Allergies
- Medical Conditions
- Medications (Names and Dosages)
- Vitamins/Supplements
- Recent Surgeries
- Emergency Contact Information

Preparation also includes deciding what degree of heroic efforts you want doctors to perform should you become comatose or lose brain function. For instance, would you want to be put on a machine that breathes for you? Do you want "life support"? We have a number of sophisticated technologies to prolong life, but the value of using them is a decision best left to patients and their families.

One way to make your intentions known is through the creation of an advance health care directive. For example, have you prepared a living will? A living will is a legal document that expresses your wishes regarding medical treatment if you no longer can make decisions for yourself. It typically describes what types of medical procedures or services you would want to receive under certain circumstances. You can describe what type of medical treatments you may or may not want, how comfortable you want to be, and whether you wish to be an organ donor. I recommend that if you are over 21, you create a living will.

It is hard to predict every medical scenario and how you might want to be treated. Therefore, I also recommend to people that they designate a durable power of attorney for health care, sometimes referred to as a health care proxy. A usual power of attorney is not sufficient because a power of attorney is no longer in force when one becomes incapacitated. That's why this type is called durable—it continues to last. The person you designate is empowered to make decisions for you regarding your care in a hospital setting or doctor's office if you become incapacitated. (They cannot make decisions for you if you are not incapacitated.) It's important to choose someone you trust, and who you feel will respect your wishes.

You might want to consult with a lawyer to help you prepare these documents. There are also many Web sites that make it easy for you to complete forms online, print them out, and get them notarized.

And please communicate your wishes to your loved ones. Too often, we neglect to mention to our family and trusted friends how much medical intervention we want if we were to become incapacitated. There's no right answer; you decide what you would want and then talk with your family. Don't let them guess, or be forced to find out about your wishes on a piece of paper. And if you choose a health care proxy, be sure your loved ones know whom you chose. I have seen too many families struggle and agonize over what to do when a parent or spouse becomes ill. Make your wishes known for everybody's benefit.

DURING THE HOSPITAL VISIT

Being in a hospital is stressful. It is easy to become scared and overwhelmed. If possible, try to have a family member or close friend with you. Not only will this make the time go faster (there's a lot of waiting around in the hospital), but it's also helpful to have another set of eyes and ears observing the care you receive. This person can be an advocate for you, especially if you're not feeling well enough to be your own advocate.

I find that patients tend to be very passive in the hospital, but it's vital to make sure you understand your diagnosis, treatment plan, and options. There will be a lot of doctors and nurses coming in and out of your room, and it can be easy to get confused. Always ask questions if you don't understand something.

I suggest to people that they write down their questions ahead of time. I also suggest that patients write down the names of the doctors who come in the room. I realize that we doctors often "breeze in" first thing in the morning while you're still groggy, go over complicated information, and then leave in 5 minutes (sometimes less!). I'm not surprised that all the information becomes a blur. Family members and friends of patients sometimes tell me they don't want to make the doctor mad by asking too many questions, but you should never be afraid to ask questions—and if the doctor doesn't answer them to your satisfaction, you can always seek out a second opinion. Sometimes doctors disagree about the treatment plan, so you might want to consider asking for someone else to review your care plan if you're uncertain about which option is best for you. You're not in the hospital to make friends; you're there to get good-quality care.

Believe it or not, you don't have to do what you are told in the hospital. You always remain in charge of your own care. But also remember that people who work in a hospital are well informed, well-intentioned, and it's their job to help you get better. The hospital staff may not always communicate with you as effectively as you'd like, and they sometimes make mistakes. As long as your mental faculties are intact and you are medically stable, you can leave the hospital at any point. You may have to sign a form that says you are leaving "against medical advice" and that you release the hospital and staff from any liability. I do not usually recommend this, since again, you are there to get better. Often it is a breakdown in communication that causes some patients to want to leave before they are considered ready to go, so speak up early and often so it does not get to that point.

AFTER THE HOSPITAL VISIT

All hospitals are required to do "discharge planning." This means that there needs to be a plan for your care once you leave the hospital. Unfortunately, not all hospitals do this well. Before you leave, you typically receive a piece of paper with the discharge diagnosis as well as the list of medications that your doctor has prescribed for you. Many times, you'll need to start a new medication, or your doctor may want you to go off of past medications or take a new dosage. It's very important to read this piece of paper carefully and keep it in a safe place. I've seen many problems occur days or weeks later because patients were confused about their medications after a hospital discharge. Don't let this happen to you. Go over each medicine—the name, the dose, what it is treating, how it should be taken, and how often to take it. Ask how long you'll need to be on each medication, if there are potential side effects you should look out for, and what to do if you miss a dose.

Nowadays it usually is the norm for a hospitalist (a physician trained in hospital care) to take care of you in the hospital, so you may not be seen by your primary care doctor. If this is the case, the physician treating you in the hospital is required to send a detailed note to your doctor explaining what was done in the hospital and why. But to be honest, this doesn't always happen. And even when it does, your primary care physician does not always receive the information about your hospitalization in a timely manner. Don't assume everyone is communicating with each other.

Try to get in touch with your primary care doctor while you are in the hospital if he or she does not already know you are there. If for some reason this does not work, definitely call the doctor's office on the day you get home. The discharge plan almost always specifies some follow-up; you want to make sure you receive it. I actually recommend to most patients that they get a copy of the physician's discharge note to keep in their own records.

CHOOSING THE RIGHT HOSPITAL

If you've read my bio on the book jacket, you will have seen that I have spent most of my career as a clinician in major academic teaching hospitals. But I'll let you in on a secret: When I've had to go to the ER for a simple problem myself, I've usually just gone to my local community hospital, and I've always received great care. My conditions were not life threatening and the hospital was pretty close to my home, so it seemed like the best choice for me.

So how do you determine what hospital is right for your needs? A teaching hospital is a hospital that is associated with a university medical school. As its name implies, it plays an important role in the clinical training of medical students and residents. In medicine, we learn by "doing." There's a common saying, "See one, do

EIGHT TIPS FOR A BETTER HOSPITAL VISIT

1 Don't hesitate to go to the hospital if you truly feel you have an emergency. You were not trained to be a doctor, and for some conditions such as stroke and heart attacks, minutes do matter.

2 If you can, call your primary care doctor before going to the emergency room. Sometimes if your symptoms are not life threatening, you can be seen in the doctor's office.

3 Be patient. The emergency department does not work on a "first-come, first-served basis." There is an elaborate triage system based on the severity of your presenting symptoms. If your symptoms are not life threatening, bring along a friend or some reading materials and expect a wait.

4 Keep all of your medications together in a small box or bag and take it with you to the hospital. It is very important for the hospital staff to know which medications you take, how much, and how often. By bringing the prescription bottles with you in a box or bag, you'll help the hospital staff to find all the information they need about your drug treatments, including who prescribed them, who filled the prescription, and how to reach them.

one, teach one." In order to make this happen, we need to be doing exams, procedures, and tests. As a result, students and residents will be involved in your care in teaching hospitals. Don't worry: Students and residents are always supervised by a senior attending physician who is ultimately responsible for your care. However, you will mostly interact with trainees.

So why bother with a teaching hospital? Some people enjoy the aspect of helping to educate future doctors. I certainly am very thankful to the thousands of patients who allowed me to be involved in their care during my years in medical school, residency, and fellowship. In addition, teaching hospitals are major referral

5 Wear and bring comfortable clothing. Items that are easy to take off and put on will prove to be very useful. Remember, you're going to the hospital, not out to dinner; try to leave valuables, such as watches and rings, at home. You don't want to risk losing them at the hospital.

6 Make sure you are carrying identification as well as your health insurance information.

7 Always keep important phone numbers handy, such as those of your close family members or your primary care doctor, in case hospital staff needs to reach them. Nowadays, we typically keep numbers stored in our phones and often we don't even know the number. Writing them down will be useful.

8 Ask everyone (staff and visitors) who comes into your room to wash their hands before they touch you. Most people do, but don't make that assumption. Germs are everywhere in a hospital and are easily spread. Simple hand washing with warm water and soap is sufficient. You don't need all the fancy sanitizers.

centers, where difficult or challenging cases are sent for evaluation and treatment. As a result, they take care of complicated and unusual cases and may have a team of experts, advanced diagnostic tools, and cutting-edge surgery and treatment techniques that other hospitals can't match. If your case is unusual or complicated, you should go to a teaching hospital.

When looking at various hospitals, it's most important to go somewhere that specializes in the treatment of your condition. For instance, if you need a knee replacement, you want to go to the surgeon and hospital that do the most knee surgeries in your area. Numerous studies have demonstrated that cardiac and stroke centers have better outcomes than the average hospital when it comes to treating heart attacks and strokes. Find out what your local hospital—whether it's a teaching hospital or not—specializes in. You might want to consider going online to find out how well your local hospital scores when it comes to treating certain medical conditions; www.hospitalcompare.hhs.gov is a great resource. It also can be worthwhile to research your doctor online. There are many free Web sites that allow patients to post reviews of their doctors. I do view these with caution, however. The reviews are not based on a statistical sample; it may not be a true representation of the doctor's practice. Nonetheless, it can provide some food for thought. It is often more useful to visit the Web site of your state's medical board to see if any disciplinary actions have been filed against a doctor or hospital.

Answers to true/false statements: False, True, False, True

APPENDIX

Screening Tests by Decade Based on Age and Gender

Age	MEN	WOMEN
40–49	Blood pressure exam every 2 years	Blood pressure exam every 2 years
	Cholesterol exam every 5 years	Cholesterol exam every 5 years, starting at age 45
	Skin exam yearly	Skin exam yearly
	Fasting plasma glucose every 3 years to check for diabetes	Pelvic exam yearly
		Pap test every 3 years
	Eye exam every year	Mammogram every 1 to 2 years; clinical breast exam yearly
	Hearing test every 10 years	
	Dental exam twice yearly	Fasting plasma glucose every 3 years to check for diabetes
		Eye exam every year
		Hearing test every 10 years
		Dental exam twice yearly
50–59	Blood pressure exam every 2 years	Baseline bone densitometry
	Cholesterol exam every 5 years	Blood pressure exam every 2 years
	Skin exam yearly	Cholesterol exam every 5 years
	PSA and digital rectal exam yearly to check for prostate cancer	Skin exam yearly
		Mammogram and clinical breast exam yearly
	Fasting plasma glucose every 3 years to check for diabetes	Pelvic exam yearly
		Pap test every 3 years
	Colorectal cancer tests:	Fasting plasma glucose every 3 years
	• Fecal occult blood test yearly	Colorectal cancer tests:
	• Flexible sigmoidoscopy every 5 years	• Fecal occult blood test yearly

(Continued)

Screening Tests by Decade Based on Age and Gender (Cont.)

Age	MEN	WOMEN
50–59 (Cont.)	• Colonoscopy every 10 years Eye exam every year Hearing test every 3 years Dental exam twice yearly	• Flexible sigmoidoscopy every 5 years • Colonoscopy every 10 years Eye exam every 3 years Hearing test every 3 years Dental exam twice yearly
60–69	Blood pressure exam every 2 years Cholesterol exam every 5 years Skin exam yearly PSA and digital rectal exam yearly to check for prostate cancer Fasting plasma glucose every 3 years to check for diabetes Colorectal cancer tests: • Fecal occult blood test yearly • Flexible sigmoidoscopy every 5 years • Colonoscopy every 10 years Eye exam every year Hearing test every 3 years Dental exam twice yearly	Blood pressure exam every 2 years Cholesterol exam every 5 years Skin exam yearly Mammogram and clinical breast exam yearly Pelvic exam yearly Pap test every 3 years Fasting plasma glucose every 3 years Thyroid-stimulating hormone test every 3 to 5 years after age 65 Colorectal cancer tests: • Fecal occult blood test yearly • Flexible sigmoidoscopy every 5 years • Colonoscopy every 10 years Eye exam every year Hearing test every 3 years Dental exam twice yearly

Screening Tests by Decade Based on Age and Gender (Cont.)

Age	MEN	WOMEN
70–79	Blood pressure exam every 2 years	Blood pressure exam every 2 years
	Cholesterol exam every 5 years	Cholesterol exam every 5 years
	Skin exam yearly	Skin exam yearly
	PSA and digital rectal exam yearly to check for prostate cancer	Mammogram and clinical breast exam yearly
		Pelvic exam yearly
	Fasting plasma glucose every 3 years to check for diabetes	Pap test every 3 years
		Fasting plasma glucose every 3 years
	Colorectal cancer tests (up to 75 years of age, afterward based on doctor recommendation):	Thyroid-stimulating hormone test every 3 to 5 years
	• Fecal occult blood test yearly	Colorectal cancer tests (up to 75 years of age, afterward based on doctor recommendation):
	• Flexible sigmoidoscopy every 5 years	• Fecal occult blood test yearly
	• Colonoscopy every 10 years	• Flexible sigmoidoscopy every 5 years
	Eye exam every year	• Colonoscopy every 10 years
	Hearing test every 3 years	Eye exam every year
	Dental exam twice yearly	Hearing test every 3 years
		Dental exam twice yearly
80–89	Blood pressure exam every 2 years	Blood pressure exam every 2 years
	Cholesterol exam every 5 years	Cholesterol exam every 5 years
	Skin exam yearly	Skin exam yearly
		Mammogram and clinical breast exam yearly

(Continued)

Screening Tests by Decade Based on Age and Gender (Cont.)

Age	MEN	WOMEN
80–89 (Cont.)	Digital rectal exam yearly to check for prostate cancer after discussion with doctor Fasting plasma glucose every 3 years to check for diabetes Eye exam every year Hearing test every 3 years Dental exam twice yearly	Pelvic exam yearly Pap test yearly Fasting plasma glucose every 3 years Thyroid-stimulating hormone test every 3 to 5 years Eye exam every year Hearing test every 3 years Dental exam twice yearly
90–99	Blood pressure exam every 2 years Cholesterol exam every 5 years Skin exam yearly Fasting plasma glucose every 3 years to check for diabetes Eye exam every year Hearing test every 3 years Dental exam twice yearly	Blood pressure exam every 2 years Cholesterol exam every 5 years Skin exam yearly Fasting plasma glucose every 3 years Thyroid-stimulating hormone test every 3 to 5 years Eye exam every year Hearing test every 3 years Dental exam twice yearly

ACKNOWLEDGMENTS

Thank you to the thousands of patients I have had the pleasure of treating over the last 15 years. Your questions and curiosity inspired me to write this book.

Thanks to my literary agent, Alan Morell, who encouraged me to submit a book proposal and leaped into action to make it a reality. His insight has been immensely valuable to me.

The team at Rodale is top notch and deserves much praise. Julie Will believed in the book concept from the get-go as well as my ability as a first-time author to get this manuscript done in record time. Marie Crousillat, Gena Smith, and Brent Gallenberger all helped to actually make this a fun process.

To my informal focus group, who read through various versions and offered constructive criticism—Allyson Saunders, Shawn Brooks, Usker Naqvi—I am grateful for your help in making this book much more informative and easy to read.

And special thanks to Dr. Beth Seltzer, who helped me organize my thoughts and provided research and commentary along the way.

Kudos to my illustrator, Judy Newhouse, who helped bring my words to life with understandable illustrations. I didn't always have the right words, but Judy always had the right pictures!

I want to thank my colleagues at Discovery for teaching me how to communicate health and medical information in both an educational and entertaining way. Eileen O'Neill, Group President of Discovery Channel and TLC, brought me on board nearly 6 years ago, and it's been an incredible journey. Sylvia Bugg, Deena Edwards, and Rosa Young all make coming to work hardly seem like work.

I am grateful to my sisters, Charlene and Jackie, who always listen to me even when I know the answers, being the consummate big sisters to their younger brother.

I need to thank my nephews, Matthew and Michael, who keep me grounded and make sure that book authorship doesn't go to my head!

I would like to thank my wife, Alisa, for her constant love and support. There were many days I was ensconced in the library, writing and rewriting the book. Thanks for all your understanding.

Finally, thanks to my mother and father, Anna Marie and John, for their unconditional love and support. You always encouraged me to pursue my dreams and provided me the support to do so. I could not ask for better parents.

NOTES

Chapter 1

[1] Dietary supplement fact sheet: Vitamin D. Office of Dietary Supplements, National Institutes of Health. Last updated November 13, 2009. http://ods.od.nih.gov/factsheets/vitamind.

[2] Morita A. Tobacco smoke and skin aging. In: Farage MA, Miller KW, Maibach HI, eds. *Textbook of Aging Skin*. Berlin: Springer-Verlag, 2010; 447.

[3] Goulden V, Stables GI, Cunliffe WJ. Prevalence of facial acne in adults. *J Am Acad Dermatol*. 1999;41:577–80.

[4] Collier CN, Harper JC, Cantrell WC, Wang W, Foster KW, Elewski BE. Prevalence of acne in adults 20 years and older. *J Am Acad Dermatol*. 2008;58(1):56–59.

Chapter 2

[1] Institute of Medicine. *Dietary Reference Intakes for Energy, Carbohydrate, Fiber, Fat, Fatty Acids, Cholesterol, Protein, and Amino Acids (Macronutrients)*. Washington, DC: The National Academies Press, 2005.

[2] Roberts SB, Dallal GE. Energy requirements and aging. *Public Health Nutrition*. 2005;8(7A):1028–36.

[3] US Department of Health and Human Services. Chapter 5: active older adults. *2008 Physical Activity Guidelines for Americans*. Last updated on October 16, 2008. http://www.health.gov/paguidelines/guidelines/Chapter5.apx.

Chapter 5

[1] Folstein M, Folstein SE, McHugh PR. Mini-mental state: a practical method for grading the cognitive state of patients for the clinician. *J Psychiatr Res* 1975;12(3): 189–98.

Chapter 11

[1] Writing Group for the Women's Health Initiative Investigators. Risks and benefits of estrogen plus progestin in healthy postmenopausal women. Principal results from the Women's Health Initiative Randomized Controlled Trial. *JAMA*. 2002;288:321–33.

[2] Mandelblatt JS, Crontin KA, Bailey S, et al. Effects of mammography screening under different screening schedules: model estimates of potential benefits and harms. *Ann Intern Med*. 2009;151:738–47.

[3] Breast cancer: detailed guide. American Cancer Society. Last revised November 16, 2010. Accessed online at http://www.cancer.org/cancer/breastcancer/detailedguide/breast-cancer-detection.

[4] http://www.cancer.org/Healthy/FindCancerEarly/WomensHealth/Non-
CancerousBreastConditions/non-cancerous-breast-conditions-a-c-s-recs-for
-early-detection.

[5] Understand your risk of heart attack. American Heart Association. Last
updated November 3, 2010. http://www.heart.org/HEARTORG/Conditions
/HeartAttack/UnderstandYourRiskofHeartAttack/Understand-Your-Risk-of
-Heart-Attack_UCM_002040_Article.jsp.

Chapter 12

[1] Testosterone therapy in adult men with androgen deficiency syndromes: an
Endocrine Society clinical practice guideline. *J Clin Endocrinol Metab.*
2010;95(6):2536–59.

[2] Calof OM, Singh AB, Lee ML, Kenny AM, Urban RJ, Tenover JL, Bhasin S.
Adverse events associated with testosterone replacement in middle-aged and
older men: a meta-analysis of randomized, placebo-controlled trials. *J Gerontol
A Biol Sci Med Sci.* 2005 Nov;60(11):1451–57.

[3] Pierorazio PM, Ferrucci L, Kettermann A, Longo DL, Metter EJ, Carter HB.
Serum testosterone is associated with aggressive prostate cancer in older men:
results from the Baltimore Longitudinal Study of Aging. *BJU Int.*
2010;105(6):824–29.

[4] American Cancer Society. *Cancer Facts & Figures 2010.* Atlanta: American
Cancer Society; 2010.

[5] American Cancer Society recommendations for early prostate cancer detection. American Cancer Society Web site. Last updated July 6, 2010. http://www
.cancer.org/Cancer/ProstateCancer/MoreInformation/ProstateCancerEarlyDe
tection/prostate-cancer-early-detection-a-c-s-recommendations.

Chapter 13

[1] Henderson AS, Jorm AF, Korten AE. Symptoms of depression and anxiety
during adult life: evidence for a decline in prevalence with age. *Psychol Med.*
1998;28:1321–28.

Chapter 14

[1] Ewing, JA. Detecting alcoholism: the CAGE questionaire. *JAMA* 1984;252:
1905–7.

RESOURCES

DERMATOLOGY

Age Page—Skin Care and Aging
www.nia.nih.gov/HealthInformation/Publications/skin.htm
This page from the National Institute on Aging provides useful information on maintaining skin health as we age. Learn the ABCDE's of skin cancer and browse the additional resources. You can read online or print the brochure.

American Academy of Dermatology
www.aad.org
This national leader in dermatology has plentiful information available on its Web site for the public to view. Just scroll over the Public tab to access information on skin conditions, testing, sun safety, and more. Take some time to download the free material. You can also find a dermatologist or free skin cancer screening in your area!

American Skin Association
www.americanskin.org
Aiming to advance research and raise awareness about skin health, the ASA has established this Web site with numerous helpful resources. The Skin Resource Center section has all the information you'll need and more.

American Society for Dermatologic Surgery
www.asds.net
Thinking about surgery? Then this is the place to go. Click on the Public tab to find easy-to-understand information on many different skin conditions. There are also explanations of treatments and surgical options. You can also locate a dermatologic surgeon near you.

Coalition of Skin Diseases
www.coalitionofskindiseases.org
An umbrella group consisting of specialized organizations for many different skin diseases, this coalition aims to advocate on behalf of patients and foster patient education. Click on Member Organizations to find organizations specializing in skin conditions such as eczema, psoriasis, and more.

Medline Plus—Skin Conditions
www.nlm.nih.gov/medlineplus/skinconditions.html
With information taken from the National Library of Medicine, this page provides thorough education on skin conditions. Learn about symptoms, diagnosis, and treatment, or view photos of common skin disorders. There are also videos and useful health check tools.

FITNESS

AARP: Health and Fitness
www.aarp.org/health/fitness
AARP offers a number of articles on the health benefits of exercise and fitness on this Web site. There are also numerous helpful tips for getting in shape and staying fit. You can find out your body mass index and what it means. You can also get discounts on fitness products and services.

American College of Sports Medicine
www.acsm.org
ACSM is a professional organization involved not only in sports medicine but also in health and exercise promotion. Under the resources menu, click on General Public to find downloadable brochures, physical activity guidelines, helpful links, and a fitness professional locator to help you find an ACSM-certified professional in your area. There is also a section dedicated to promoting fitness in seniors.

HelpGuide.org: Senior Exercise and Fitness
www.helpguide.org/life/senior_fitness_sports.htm
The nonprofit HelpGuide offers valuable advice for getting fit and healthy through this Web page. It presents myths about exercise, tips for getting started safely, advice on creating a balanced exercise plan, and much more.

International Council on Active Aging
www.icaa.cc
This network of more than 8,000 organizations is committed to promoting health and fitness throughout the aging process. Click on the Consumer Section and you will find an abundance of resources, such as a thorough guide to getting started, information on walking, a foot health guide, and much more. Click on How to Choose a Facility to find directories of age-friendly health clubs, fitness centers, and personal trainers.

National Blueprint: Increasing Physical Activity among Adults Aged 50 and Older
www.agingblueprint.org
This project by the Active Aging Partnership—a coalition of organizations including AARP, American Geriatrics Society, American College of Sports Medicine, National Center for Aging, and more—aims to increase physical activity in older adults. You can view the blueprint on this Web site as well as read other informative articles on staying fit in the older years.

National Center on Physical Activity and Disability
www.ncpad.org
This very helpful Web site is loaded with resources for those whose age or diseases have left them feeling discouraged about exercising. There are various articles on different modes of exercise, how to keep fit despite having different diseases, how exercise can benefit the treatment of diseases, and much more. Have a look at the Videos section, which contains many helpful demonstrations and exercise programs.

NIHSeniorHealth: Exercise and Physical Activity for Older Adults

www.nihseniorhealth.gov/exerciseforolderadults/toc.html

The National Institutes of Health presents a guide to exercise directed to the senior population. The Web site has a simple layout and is easy to navigate, with adjustable text size and audio narration capability. There is advice on the benefits of exercise, tips for getting started, exercises to try, instructional videos, and more.

President's Council on Fitness, Sports, and Nutrition

www.fitness.gov

This committee of volunteer citizens serves to advise the government on healthy and active lifestyles. Here you can find the federal guidelines for diet and exercise. There are also photos, a recipe finder, and videos. You can also find out about the President's Challenge and President's Active Lifestyle Award.

GI PROBLEMS

American College of Gastroenterology

www.acg.gi.org

This professional organization for gastroenterologists has many patient education resources available. Under the Patients tab, you will find articles spanning the range of gastrointestinal conditions. There are also brochures, podcasts, and other interactive tools. You can even find a GI or liver specialist in your area.

American Gastroenterological Association

www.gastro.org

This international professional organization for physicians has made plenty of patient resources available under the Patient Center menu. You can learn about gastroenterology in general or choose articles on specific diseases and conditions. There is also a section on procedures that provides guidance on how to prepare for procedures such as endoscopies and what to expect from them. The Diet and Medication section covers the consequences that food and drugs can have on your GI tract.

American Liver Foundation

www.liverfoundation.org

The American Liver Foundation aims to promote education about liver diseases. The pull-down menu on the home page allows you to select from a vast range of liver disease topics. You can also find a liver specialist near you or learn about support programs. The foundation also organizes a number of events and programs, such as walks, culinary galas, and musical events, to raise awareness or funds for research.

International Foundation for Functional Gastrointestinal Disorders

www.iffgd.org

This nonprofit organization aims to inform and support those who suffer from GI disorders. It is very active in advocacy, and these efforts are prominently displayed on its Web site. There is also a section on GI Disorders and a Library tab with current publications and other helpful reading. You can also find links to its disease-specific pages.

National Cancer Institute: Colon and Rectal Cancer

www.cancer.gov/cancertopics/types/colon-and-rectal

The National Cancer Institute maintains this page that contains information on two common GI cancers. There are helpful sections on prevention, causes, treatment, screening and testing, statistics, and much more. There are also online booklets and up-to-date reports on the most current cancer research.

National Digestive Diseases Information Clearinghouse

www.digestive.niddk.nih.gov/

This clearinghouse is an information dissemination service of the National Institute of Diabetes and Digestive and Kidney Diseases, part of the National Institutes of Health. Its goal is to make information about digestive diseases available to patients and the general public. Here you can find national statistics, an A-to-Z list of articles on digestive diseases, a series on awareness and prevention, and much more.

National Pancreas Foundation

www.pancreasfoundation.org

This organization's mission is to support research and education of pancreatic disease. There is in-depth information on pancreatitis and pancreatic cancer in the appropriate menus, even covering subjects such as alternative therapies and nutrition advice. Click on the Healthy Lifestyle Guide for articles full of tips on how to stay healthy and prevent pancreatic disease.

HEARING

Academy of Doctors of Audiology

www.audiologist.org

The Academy of Doctors of Audiology is a professional organization that offers hearing resources for patients and the public. Just click on the Patients tab and you'll find a vast network of specialized hearing organizations and other useful tools. The patient FAQ section is very helpful, and the audiologist directory can help you locate a hearing professional.

American Academy of Otolaryngology—Head and Neck Surgery

www.entnet.org

Commonly known as ENTs, otolaryngologists are doctors who specialize in ear, nose, and throat health. Click on the Health Information tab to go to the patient education section. There you will find a number of articles on a wide range of ear health topics. You can also use the Find an ENT feature to learn about ear doctors in your area.

Better Hearing Institute

www.betterhearing.org

BHI works to promote hearing health and fight the stigma associated with hearing loss. Find information on a wealth of hearing topics, read the blog, or post in the discussion forums. The Web site also posts profiles from Hollywood celebrities about their struggles with hearing loss. Try out the hearing loss simulator and the online hearing test!

Deafness Research Foundation

www.drf.org

DRF aims to promote hearing health by supporting research and engaging in advocacy. At their Web site, you can read about hearing health programs and find a hearing professional in your area. Be sure to check out Hearing Health *magazine by clicking on the link at the top of the page. It has excellent articles and resources for the general public.*

Hear-It

www.hear-it.org

This European nonprofit is committed to circulating up-to-date scientific information on hearing health. There is a wealth of facts, statistics, and articles to teach you all about protecting your hearing, how to treat hearing loss, and more. Click on the Interactive tab for sound files, an online hearing test, hearing questionnaires, and other great, interactive resources.

How's Your Hearing?

www.howsyourhearing.org

This Web site by the American Academy of Audiology presents helpful resources that are easy to understand. You can learn about hearing loss, hearing aids, aural rehabilitation, and more. You can also search for an audiologist in your area. All content is contributed by professional audiologists and hearing researchers.

National Institute on Aging

www.nia.nih.gov

Also a branch of the National Institutes of Health, the NIA provides information not only about aging but also specifically on health issues related to hearing. Click on the Health tab to browse a number of categories. You can sign up for e-mail alerts or browse their vast directory of affiliated professional organizations.

National Institute on Deafness and Other Communication Disorders

www.nidcd.nih.gov

NIDCD is a branch of the National Institutes of Health that focuses on hearing and communication issues. There is an A-to-Z index of hearing-related topics as well as statistics on hearing health. You can order free information, learn about hearing protection, or try the Distorted Tunes Test.

MEMORY

Alzheimer's Association

www.alz.org

This leading nonprofit for Alzheimer's advocacy and support provides plentiful resources for education and awareness of Alzheimer's. You can read up on the basics or take a virtual tour of the brain! There is also a great interactive course to teach you how to identify the signs of Alzheimer's disease.

FamilyDoctor.Org: Memory Loss with Aging

http://familydoctor.org/online/famdocen/home/seniors/common-older/124.html

This resource from the American Academy of Family Physicians answers common questions about memory loss in simple, easy-to-understand language. You can find tips on preserving memory and how to tell whether your memory loss is related to aging.

HelpGuide.Org: How to Improve Your Memory

http://helpguide.org/life/improving_memory.htm

HelpGuide is a nonprofit whose mission is to help the public learn about making healthy choices. This useful list of tips and exercises can help you preserve or improve your memory and learn more about how memory works. Be sure to take a look at the Seniors and Aging section on the side menu; the Alzheimer's/Dementia section provides further information on memory loss.

Medline PLUS: Dementia

www.nlm.nih.gov/medlineplus/dementia.html

Medline's guide to dementia provides up-to-date information on mental health and memory loss in the elderly. All information comes from the National Library of Medicine. There are sections for updates on the latest research, printable handouts, helpful overviews, and more. Be sure to check out the videos section as well!

Mental Health and Aging

www.mhaging.org

MH&A provides a guide for older adults to understand how to preserve their mental health, how to know if their mental health is suffering, and what kinds of treatments are available. This organization strongly supports advocacy.

NYU Medical Center: Age-Associated Memory Impairment

www.med.nyu.edu/adc/forpatients/memory.html

NYU Medical Center maintains a thorough Web page to teach the public about memory changes with aging. You can learn about diagnosis, causes, treatment options, and more!

University of Michigan: Memory and Aging

www.med.umich.edu/1libr/aha/ummemory.htm

This Web page from the University of Michigan Health System describes aging-related memory changes in Q&A format. The information is easy to understand and comes from a trusted university source. The section for further reading has numerous useful articles.

MEN'S HEALTH

Centers for Disease Control and Prevention—Men's Health

www.cdc.gov/men

This Web site organizes all of the information available from this prominent government research center. You can test your knowledge, read about topics from A to Z, or browse tips for a healthy life. It is frequently updated to reflect the latest research and news in men's health.

FamilyDoctor.org—Men's Health

http://familydoctor.org/online/famdocen/home/men.html

FamilyDoctor.org is a patient information resource by the American Academy of Family Physicians, the foremost organization for family medicine. There is information on many general health topics but also specific sections such as prostate health, reproductive health, fatherhood, and more.

Medline Plus: Men's Health

www.nlm.nih.gov/medlineplus/menshealth.html

This section, designed by the National Institutes of Health, focuses specifically on men's health. Produced by the National Library of Medicine, this site contains information on countless health topics for men. There are sections for the latest news, diagnosis, treatment, prevention, nutrition, and much more!

Men's Health Network

www.menshealthnetwork.org

This national nonprofit organization strives to foster health care education for men and increase their physical and mental health. Browse the Library and Resource Center tabs to find loads of information on just about any health topic. The "Blueprint for Men's Health" guide is particularly useful!

MENTAL HEALTH

Mental Health America

www.mentalhealthamerica.net

If you're looking for information on mental health advocacy, this is one of the places to go. MHA's network of mental health patients, their families and friends, and others is dedicated to bringing mental health issues to the forefront. You can also find information on a wide range of mental health issues as well as find treatment and support groups and get help paying for prescriptions.

Mental Health and Aging

www.mhaging.org

MH&A provides a guide for older adults to understand how to preserve their mental health, how to know if their mental health is suffering, and what kinds of treatments are available. This organization also strongly supports advocacy.

MentalHelp.net

www.mentalhelp.net

With a host of physicians, psychologists, social workers, and more contributing content to this Web site, it is a convenient place to get educated on a range of mental health topics. There are discussion forums, blogs, articles, videos, and other media, all serving to provide information to the general public. You can also post a question for a psychiatrist to answer online.

National Alliance on Mental Illness

www.nami.org

NAMI has an extensive collection of information on mental illnesses, medications, and support programs. Perhaps most notable are its grassroots efforts for advocacy and its work to shine the spotlight on improving mental health. Go "old school" and call their toll-free helpline or look for a local chapter!

National Coalition on Mental Health and Aging

www.ncmha.org

NCMHA is composed of professional, consumer, and governmental organizations focused on mental health issues. It encourages advocacy and maintains directories of information on mental health.

National Institutes of Mental Health

www.nimh.nih.gov

NIMH is a division of the National Institutes of Health. This site provides loads of information on mental health conditions and how to get help. There are also facts and statistics and information on the latest mental health research.

PAIN

American Academy of Pain Medicine

www.painmed.org

This professional organization for pain doctors has made much information available online for patients. Just click on Patient Center from the home page and you will find facts about pain, tips to prevent drug abuse, and informative videos. You can also find a pain management doctor in your area.

American Academy of Physical Medicine and Rehabilitation

www.aapmr.org

This professional organization for physicians makes many pain resources available. There is a lot of useful information available under Conditions and Treatment. You can also find a physician who specializes in physical medicine and rehabilitation for nonsurgical approaches to treating your pain.

American Chronic Pain Association

www.theacpa.org

This advocacy organization offers education in pain management skills and support groups in many countries. On their Web site, there is an A-to-Z listing on pain conditions, a guide to medications and treatments, and a rich selection of helpful tools. Click on Pain Management Tools to access videos, surveys, links, tips for going to the emergency room, and much more.

American Pain Foundation

www.painfoundation.org

APF is a nonprofit whose goal is to provide support and advocacy for those affected by pain. You can read about pain conditions, living with pain, and much more. The Pain Resource Locator is a particularly useful feature that connects patients with disease-specific support organizations.

Arthritis Foundation
www.arthritis.org
The Arthritis Foundation is the only national nonprofit organization supporting all forms of arthritis. Click on the Diseases tab to access the Disease Center, Surgery Center, Pain Center, Q&A, and other helpful sections. There is also information on alternative therapies and a message board so that you can discuss arthritis pain with other patients. Also, take a look at the Events & Programs tab to find out about fund-raisers and events that support arthritis and pain research and treatment.

National Institutes of Neurological Disorders and Stroke: Chronic Pain
www.ninds.nih.gov/disorders/chronic_pain/chronic_pain.htm
This National Institutes of Health branch maintains a wide range of publications on pain management as well as a helpful Q&A on chronic pain. There are also sections for the latest news and links to professional organizations dedicated to pain management.

National Pain Foundation
www.nationalpainfoundation.org
NPF is a nonprofit that aims to educate the public about pain management. There is a wide range of resources here centered on pain management, including a community discussion forum, latest news, diseases and conditions directory, and much more. For information relevant to aging, click on the Living tab, then choose Seniors and Pain from the menu.

PATIENT SAFETY

Clean Hands Save Lives
www.cleanhandssavelives.org
This site from the State of Pennsylvania focuses on hand-washing hygiene as an important strategy in reducing hospital-acquired infections. You can find explanations of symptoms, risk factors, causes, and more. There are also guides for how to minimize infection at home or in the hospital and what to ask your doctor to make sure you have the safest experience possible.

Consumers Advancing Patient Safety
www.patientsafety.org
CAPS seeks to promote a partnership between consumers and health care providers that would improve quality of care. At this Web site, you can learn about becoming a member or share your own story about patient safety. Click on the Resources heading to find a number of articles on different patient safety topics, such as infection control, medication safety, communication, anesthesia safety, and much more. There are also informative and entertaining videos to watch.

Medline PLUS: Patient Safety

www.nlm.nih.gov/medlineplus/patientsafety.html

The National Institutes of Health presents this informative Web page on patient safety, with information from the National Library of Medicine. You can find the latest news on hospital-acquired infections, for example, or read up on tips to keep yourself safe at your next hospital visit. There are also convenient printable handouts and videos on preventing errors in your treatment.

National Center for Patient Safety

www.patientsafety.gov

This federal resource offers background information, fact sheets, tips, tools, and much more on a wide range of patient safety topics, such as hand washing and falls. Visit the Newsroom section to stay updated on the latest developments in patient safety. There are also safety checklists and a helpful FAQ section.

National Patient Safety Foundation

www.npsf.org

NPSF seeks to improve patient safety by educating the general public. Click on the Patients and Families tab to find loads of information on how to keep safe and avoid medical errors. You can also share this information with your family so that they can be prepared if the occasion arises. There is a helpful forum for discussion and information on Patient Safety Awareness Week.

Prevent Infection

www.preventinfection.org

This Web site is an initiative of the Association for Professionals in Infection Control and Epidemiology, the Centers for Disease Control and Prevention, and other organizations and provides information on patient safety through infection prevention. The Prevention Central tab provides loads of background information on common infections, such as food-borne infections and skin infections. The Resources tab contains articles, brochures, and more helpful links.

Safe Care Campaign

www.safecarecampaign.org

This humanitarian organization aims to not only educate the public on patient safety but also to work with hospitals and health care providers to ensure that safety standards are effective. The site is full of valuable resources, from the In the News section to the Infection Facts section and more. The For Patients section has many videos and printable brochures on various safety topics, such as MRSA infection, hand washing, catheter safety, ventilator safety, and more.

World Health Organization: Patient Safety

www.who.int/patientsafety/en

WHO, the international health-coordinating authority of the United Nations, maintains this useful Web page on patient safety. This resource provides information on a global scale, with reports and articles from around the world as well as interviews with global health care leaders. The News and Events section can help keep you abreast of the latest issues in patient safety, such as emerging infections and pandemics.

SEX AND ROMANCE

Medline Plus—Erectile Dysfunction

www.nlm.nih.gov/medlineplus/erectiledysfunction.html

Medline's specialized section for erectile dysfunction provides all the most current information. Read about statistics, diagnosis, and treatment. There's also an informative interactive tutorial!

Medline Plus—Sexual Health

www.nlm.nih.gov/medlineplus/sexualhealth.html

This resource provides overviews, latest news, and much more on sexual health. The information is drawn from the National Library of Medicine, so you know that it is thorough. There is even a special section dedicated to seniors!

Sex Health Matters

www.sexhealthmatters.org

Run by the Sexual Medicine Society of North America, this patient education Web site offers practical information on sexual health. There are helpful videos, a blog, and a news section.

SexualMed.org

www.sexualmed.org

This Web site is operated by the nonprofit Institute for Sexual Medicine. It provides articles on sexual health issues for men and women, as well as diagnostic tests and treatment. You can discuss your problems in the community forums or post a question to an expert. You can also find a sexual health specialist in your area.

Women's Health—Sexual Health

www.womenshealth.gov/aging/sexual-health

This government source provides lots of excellent information in this section dedicated specifically to sexual health and aging. Browse through the fact sheets and other resources to learn about how to keep your sex life healthy.

SLEEP

American Psychological Association

www.apa.org

As the foremost professional organization for psychology, the APA offers resources that not only address sleep disorders but also other psychological conditions that accompany them. Browse the broad directory of topics and read through articles or the latest headlines. You can also find a psychologist near you.

American Sleep Apnea Association

www.sleepapnea.org

Visit this site to learn about sleep apnea. There is a forum for discussion with other patients and a nationwide directory of support groups. Take some time to look through the large directory of sleep services and products. You can also check your Snore Score!

American Sleep Association
www.sleepassociation.org
The American Sleep Association is composed of physicians and scientists specializing in sleep medicine. Their Web site contains a helpful patient education section with an A-to-Z encyclopedia of sleep disorders, downloadable patient handouts and questionnaires, as well as a directory of sleep products and services. You can also look for a sleep lab in your area.

National Sleep Foundation
www.sleepfoundation.org
National Sleep Foundation is a nonprofit organization that seeks to educate the public about sleep health and advocate for its importance to the government. Read up on hot topics, watch videos, sign up for the newsletter, or ask the expert. You can also find sleep professionals in your area and browse an extensive audio library.

SleepCenters.org
www.sleepcenters.org
Looking for a sleep center near you? This is a site to visit. This Web site is run by the American Academy of Sleep Medicine and serves as a nationwide directory of accredited sleep centers.

SleepEducation.com
www.sleepeducation.com
This site was established by the American Academy of Sleep Medicine to serve as a way to educate the public. You can find abundant information on any sleep topic written by top professionals. Use the online sleep evaluation tools, pose a question to a sleep specialist, and study treatment options.

SUBSTANCE ABUSE

Age Page: Alcohol Use in Older People
www.nia.nih.gov/healthinformation/publications/alcohol.htm
The National Institute on Aging provides this thorough resource on alcohol abuse. There are clearly written sections on alcohol and medications, how to know when you're drinking too much, and getting help. There is also a directory of professional organizations to help with substance abuse and treatment.

Aging in the Know: Substance Abuse
www.healthinaging.org/agingintheknow/chapters_ch_trial.asp?ch=36
This chapter from "Aging in the Know"—an expert-run information resource by the American Geriatrics Society Foundation for Healthy Aging—discusses substance abuse at length. You can learn about causes, signs, treatment, and more.

Center for Healthy Aging: Substance Abuse
www.healthyagingprograms.org/content.asp?sectionid=71
This collection of resources includes fact sheets, brochures, tests, learning modules, tool

kits, and more. All are designed to help you learn more about alcohol or drug abuse. With these helpful tools, you can be prepared to identify and prevent substance abuse.

National Institute on Alcohol Abuse and Alcoholism
www.niaaa.nih.gov
A branch of the National Institutes of Health, NIAAA focuses specifically on alcohol abuse. Click on the Publications tab to find a wealth of fact sheets, posters, brochures, and more, all for free. There is also a helpful listing of frequently asked questions meant specifically for the general public.

Recovery Connection: Senior Citizen Drug Rehab
www.recoveryconnection.org/senior-citizen-drug-rehab.php
Visit this vast resource to learn all about elderly substance abuse. There is a hotline number you can call as well as a directory of support groups. You can also find treatment centers in your state and sober living homes. There is also a free downloadable guide for friends and family.

Seniors in Sobriety
www.seniorsinsobriety.org/index.htm
Created to help senior alcoholics help other senior alcoholics achieve sobriety together, this organization maintains a helpful Web site with information on substance abuse and how to identify it. You can find out about SIS conferences and meetings in your area.

Substance Abuse and Mental Health Services Administration
www.oas.samhsa.gov/aging.cfm
This government resource provides a number of reports on substance abuse in older adults. It has compiled data from different research organizations to provide updated statistics and projections for the future of substance abuse treatment in the aging population.

UROLOGY

American Geriatric Society Foundation—Bladder Control Problems
www.healthinaging.org/public_education/bladder_control.php
AGS's Health in Aging project seeks to educate the aging patient on a variety of topics. This section is dedicated to bladder control and urinary health. Take some time to browse the many informative items posted here, such as the explanations of various treatments.

American Urological Association Foundation
www.urologyhealth.org
As the patient education branch of the leading national organization for urology, this foundation has provided many resources for your benefit on its Web site. Click on the Patient Education tab to access a wealth of information written and reviewed by expert

urologists. You can participate in webinars or view previous webinars that have been posted. You can also find a urologist in your area.

Know Your Stats

www.knowyourstats.org

This joint program between the American Urological Association Foundation and the National Football League aims to raise awareness about prostate health. There are numerous good resources here, including a Myths and Facts section. You can also find an event that hosts free screenings in your area. Be sure to check out the online risk calculator tool to find your risk for developing prostate cancer.

MyPelvicHealth.org

www.mypelvichealth.org

This is a patient education initiative from the American Urogynecologic Society Foundation that aims to teach women about pelvic disorders such as urinary incontinence. You can find an excellent range of information on bladder health here. Click on Tools for Patients to access interactive quizzes, exercises, and a bladder diary.

National Association for Continence

www.nafc.org

Dedicated to improving the quality of life of people with incontinence, NAFC has made its Web site a helpful resource for the average patient looking to learn more. Take the diagnostic quiz to assess your continence, and learn about common diagnostic tests that your doctor may use. There is also an online store with helpful products for bladder health and more.

National Kidney and Urologic Diseases Information Clearinghouse

www.kidney.niddk.nih.gov

As a subsection of the National Institutes of Health, this service provides important statistics and information on the range of kidney and urologic diseases. There is an A-to-Z list of topics as well as helpful guidance on preventing urologic diseases.

VISION

AgingEye

www.agingeye.net

Eye diseases common in aging are at the focus of this Web site. Read about numerous diseases, what their symptoms are, how they are diagnosed, and how they are treated. There are also vision myths and online vision tests. All content is written by ophthalmologists.

EyeCare America

www.eyecareamerica.org

EyeCare America is a public service foundation of the American Academy of Oph-

thalmology that provides free educational materials and facilitates access to eye care. Visit this Web site to learn about the parts of the eye, diseases and conditions, and treatment methods. There are also interactive tools such as videos and eye disease simulators. You can even see if you qualify for a free eye exam. Content is also available in Spanish.

EyeSmart

www.geteyesmart.org

EyeSmart is a campaign by the American Academy of Ophthalmology to raise awareness about eye health. It has excellent resources for patients and the general public, like information on diseases and conditions, explanations of treatment procedures, and tips for keeping your eyes healthy. There is even a feature that allows you to post a question to an eye doctor or find an eye doctor in your area.

EyeWiki

http://eyewiki.aao.org

EyeWiki is a rich resource for eye health information written not just by ophthalmologists but also by doctors of many fields. It is frequently updated with new topic entries.

National Eye Institute

www.nei.nih.gov

As a division of the National Institutes of Health, the NEI provides nationwide statistics on eye disease. The Eye Health Information section is particularly helpful, featuring an A-to-Z list of eye diseases and disorders. Content is also available in Spanish.

Prevent Blindness America

www.preventblindness.org

PBA aims to provide vision education to all ages. This Web site provides resources for research, advocacy, vision screening, and more. A nice feature is the collection of eye tests that you can do in your own home.

WebMD Eye Health Center

www.webmd.com/eye-health

The Eye Health Center at WebMD is packed with information on common eye problems and how to treat them. There are pictures and slide shows for you to view. The site also features sections for the latest headlines and top stories in eye care to keep you up to date.

Women's Eye Health.org

www.womenseyehealth.org

Citing that two-thirds of blindness and visual impairment worldwide occur in women, this Web site is dedicated to informing women about eye health. There are sections on prevention and care, statistics, eye basics, and more. Be sure to check out the wide range of printable brochures!

WOMEN'S HEALTH

American Congress of Obstetricians and Gynecologists
www.acog.org
Click on the ACOG Patient Page to be directed to a rich resource of pamphlets and information. The Find an Ob-Gyn feature is quite helpful if you're looking for a doctor.

Centers for Disease Control and Prevention—Women's Health
www.cdc.gov/women
This Web site organizes all the information available from the CDC. You can test your knowledge, read about topics from A to Z, or browse tips for a healthy life. It is frequently updated to reflect the latest research and news in women's health. Take a break from reading and try the podcasts and snapshots!

Mayo Clinic—Women's Health
www.mayoclinic.com/health/womens-health/MY00379
Mayo Clinic is one of the most respected academic health centers in the country. The women's health section of this Web site offers many resources for learning about a broad range of topics. Check out the Multimedia and Expert Answers tabs!

Medline Plus: Women's Health
www.nlm.nih.gov/medlineplus/womenshealth.html
This section, created by the National Institutes of Health, focuses specifically on women's health. Produced by the National Library of Medicine, this site contains information on countless health topics for women. There are sections for the latest news, diagnosis, treatment, prevention, nutrition, and much more!

MyPelvicHealth.org
www.mypelvichealth.org
This is a patient education initiative from the American Urogynecologic Society Foundation that aims to teach women about pelvic disorders like urinary incontinence. You can find an excellent range of information on bladder health. Click on Tools for Patients to access interactive quizzes, exercises, and a bladder diary.

National Women's Health Information Center
www.womenshealth.gov
As the federal government's source for women's health information, this site offers information on national statistics, health topics, health organizations, and more. There is also a section on health campaigns, showcasing some of the efforts to promote education on important topics such as healthy eating and heart health.

North American Menopause Society
www.menopause.org/Consumers.aspx
This nonprofit organization aims to promote women's health through understanding menopause. Click on the For Consumers tab to access their patient resources. You can learn all about combating menopause and even find a menopause specialist in your area.

INDEX

Boldface page references indicate illustrations. Underscored references indicate tables or boxed text.

H

Hair, 12–14, **13**, <u>14</u>, 31–33
Healing, slow or lacking, 10, 25
Health care proxy, 228–29
Hearing aids, 123
Hearing loss, 109–23. *See also* Ears
  age-related, 111–12
  dizziness with, <u>117</u>, 120–22
  improving hearing after, 123
  loud sounds causing, 112–14
  measurements for loudness, 112–13,
    <u>113</u>
  medications causing, 118
  normal (presbycusis), 111
  normal and not normal signs, <u>117</u>
  questions for evaluating, 114–15
  rapid or sudden, 112
  risk factors for, 112
  temporary, 109–10
  tests for, 115–17
  tips for preventing, <u>121</u>
  types of, 114
Heartburn, 53
Heart disease, 72, 154, 168, 170, 176–81
Height, decrease with age, <u>44</u>, 45–46
Helicobacter pylori (H. pylori), 62
Herpes zoster (shingles), 19–20, **20**
Hip replacement surgery, <u>144–45</u>,
    146–47
HIV, 160–61
Hormone replacement therapy (HRT),
    168–69, 171
Horny goat weed, 160
Hospital visits, 225–34
  after, 230–31
  before, 226–29
  choosing a hospital, 231–34
  during, 229–30
  tips for, <u>232–33</u>
Hot flashes, 165, 170, <u>182–83</u>
Hyaluronic acid, 4, 29
Hypodermis, **3**, 4, 6
Hypothalamic-pituitary-testicular axis,
    191
Hypothalamus, 127, 190

I

Impacted cerumen, 118
Incontinence, 65–67, 71–73
Insomnia, 130. *See also* Sleep
Intelligence, aging and, 80–81
Iris, **95**, 96
Itchiness, 16

J

Joint pain, 144–48, <u>144–45</u>

K

Kegels, 75–76
Keratinocytes, 3
Kidney disease, 67
Kidneys, 68–69, **68**
Kinetin, 28
Knee replacement, <u>144–45</u>, 146–47

L

Large intestine, **51**, 52, 55
L-arginine, 159–60
Laser treatments for hair loss, 32
Late-onset hypogonadism (LOH), 188
Laxatives, 56
Lens of eye, **95**, 97
Leydig cells, 190
Libido, low, 153–54
Liver, **51**, 52
Liver disease, 170
Liver spots, 11, **11**
Living will, 228
Luteinizing hormone (LH), 190

M

Maca, 160
Macula, **95**, 97
Macular degeneration, 105–7, **105**, <u>106–7</u>
Male menopause, 187–88, <u>202</u>
Male pattern baldness, 12–13, **13**
Mammograms, 172–73
Medications
  abuse of, 217–19, <u>222–23</u>
  arthritis, 145
  conditions due to, 82, 83, 118, 138,
    154–55, 215
  constipation, 56
  erectile dysfunction, 155–58, 193
  growth hormone, 30, 48–49
  pain relief, 142–43
  sleep aids, 138–39
  ulcer, 63
  urinary problem, 76
Melanocytes, 4
Melanoma, 24
Memory, 79, <u>84</u>, <u>89</u>
Memory loss, 81–93
  Alzheimer's, 84, 85–86, <u>90–91</u>, 92–93
  caregivers' role with, 92–93
  case study, <u>90–91</u>
  danger signs, 84–85
  increase with age, 81–82
  during menopause, 167
  normal and not normal, <u>84</u>
  preventing, 89–92
  reversible causes of, 82–83
  tests and screenings for, 86–88, 92